CAROTID ENDARTERECTOMY

CAROTID ENDARTERECTOMY

Principles and Technique

Second Edition

CHRISTOPHER M. LOFTUS

Temple University
Philadelphia, Pennsylvania, U.S.A.

informa
healthcare

New York   London

Informa Healthcare USA, Inc.
270 Madison Avenue
New York, NY 10016

© 2007 by Informa Healthcare USA, Inc.
Informa Healthcare is an Informa business

No claim to original U.S. Government works
Printed in the United States of America on acid-free paper
10 9 8 7 6 5 4 3 2 1

International Standard Book Number-10: 0-8247-2832-7 (Hardcover)
International Standard Book Number-13: 978-0-8247-2832-8 (Hardcover)

This book contains information obtained from authentic and highly regarded sources. Reprinted material is quoted with permission, and sources are indicated. A wide variety of references are listed. Reasonable efforts have been made to publish reliable data and information, but the author and the publisher cannot assume responsibility for the validity of all materials or for the consequences of their use.

Library of Congress Cataloging-in-Publication Data

Loftus, Christopher M.
   Carotid endarterectomy : principles and technique / by Christopher M. Loftus.--2nd ed.
      p. ; cm.
   Includes bibliographical references and index.
   ISBN-13: 978-0-8247-2832-8 (hardcover : alk. paper)
   ISBN-10: 0-8247-2832-7 (hardcover : alk. paper)
   1. Carotid artery--Surgery. 2. Enarterectomy. I. Title.
   [DNLM: 1. Endarterectomy, Carotid--methods--Atlases. 2. Carotid Artery Diseases--surgery--Atlases. 3. Endarterectomy, Carotid--Atlases. WG 17 L829c 2006]
RD598.6.L64 2006
617.4'13--dc22
                                        2006043872

Visit the Informa Web site at
www.informa.com

and the Informa Healthcare Web site at
www.informahealthcare.com

This book is dedicated to the memory of my father,
Angel N. Miranda, M.D.,
who lived to see the first edition, but not the second one.

Preface to the Second Edition

It is a privilege to be able to write a second preface for a new edition of *Carotid Endarterectomy: Principles and Technique,* twelve years after I wrote the orginal one. As I had predicted in that first preface, the scientific and epidemiologic universe surrounding carotid artery surgery has changed dramatically—and for the better, for both surgeons and patients—during this time.

Of course I have moved on in the academic world since 1994, first to assume the Harry Wilkins Chair of Neurosurgery at the University of Oklahoma in 1997 and then in 2004 to become Professor and Chairman of the Department of Neurosurgery at Temple University in Philadelphia. Perhaps the only constant is my ongoing fascination with the scientific background and technical performance of carotid artery surgery. I have been fortunate to have outstanding neurology and vascular surgery colleagues at both of these institutions, as I had at Iowa when the first edition was published.

We know so much more now than we did in 1994 about the propriety of carotid reconstruction based on quality data from credible investigators around the world. For asymptomatic disease the ACST results have reinforced the strong data from ACAS, and validate a surgical option in stroke prevention for these patients. The NASCET data, the early iteration of which we discussed in the first edition, has been expanded to validate a surgical option for 50% or greater symptomatic stenosis, data which correlate well with ECST and VASST.

The endovascular universe has changed as well. Quality devices, with protected stenting, now offer a viable and seemingly enduring treatment option for patients with carotid disease who have co-morbidities that preclude a surgical approach. Data regarding equivalency of endovascular treatment for routine carotid patients do not yet exist, except perhaps for SAPPHIRE-studied high-risk patients, and I implore the reader to study that data carefully, as discussed in Chapter 1, and draw your own conclusions. Clearly there will be new high-quality cooperative trials comparing endovascular and surgical approaches, and thoughtful surgeons will need to study these data carefully, and potentially revise their practice patterns, if the data justify a change at some future time.

The reader will note that we have a new publisher. The publishing rights for *Carotid Artery Surgery: Principles and Technique* were sold to Marcel Dekker, Inc. several years ago, and as part of that transfer I agreed to begin work on this second edition. As time passed Marcel Dekker was absorbed into Informa Healthcare U.S.A., who have completed the task with me. They have proved to be wonderful partners, professional, organized, and efficient, and I hope the reader will find that this book justifies my confidence in them, and theirs in me. In particular, I am indebted to Geoff Greenwood in England, who made the initial contact and directed the project, Dana Bigelow in New York, who collated and assimilated all the new materials with me, and Joanne Jay at The Egerton Group Ltd., who took charge of production.

This book, then, represents twelve years additional experience on my part with carotid surgery. I have significantly expanded and updated the didactic material in Chapter 1, and I feel it is quite current. There are many more cases and interesting examples of anatomical variants, and an expanded section on complications. I retained much of the old material from the first edition, substituted a few new photographs when I thought they could be improved upon, but mostly added new material from the storehouse of clinical material that I have been accumulating in the intervening decade (plus).

As in the first edition I hope the readers find this information useful, educational, and valid, and that in some small way it advances our knowledge of carotid surgical philosophy and technique. I have been most gratified at the positive worldwide reception that was afforded to the first edition, and based on that it has been my privilege to train surgeons from many international centers who have come to visit and observe. It is my earnest hope that this current offering, which to my mind really offers much greater depth and experience, will prove to be useful to practicing surgeons as well.

Carotid surgery, performed by skilled surgeons with quantifiable results, prevents stroke in asymptomatic and symptomatic patients. The facts are unimpeachable. Our challenge now is to continually refine the techniques to ensure the greatest possible margins of safety, and to educate surgeons around the world to ensure uniform standards of care for all deserving patients.

Christopher M. Loftus

Contents

CHAPTER 1

Historical Perspective on Carotid Reconstruction

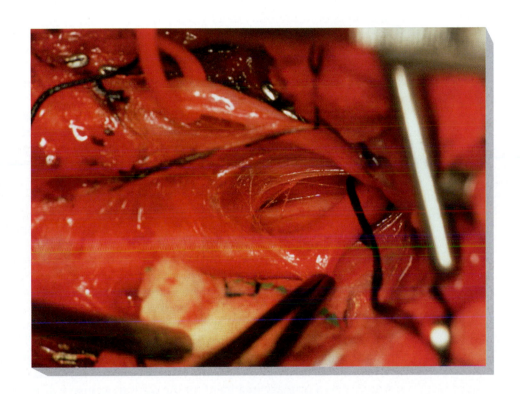

The first mention of carotid artery surgery occurred in 1793 and is credited to Hebenstreit, who performed a carotid artery ligation for carotid injury (1). However, the first deliberate ligation of the carotid artery occurred in 1798 and was performed by John Abernathy (2). The ligation was performed on a patient whose carotid artery had been torn by the horn of a cow. In 1805, Sir Astley Cooper performed a cervical carotid ligation for treatment of a cervical carotid aneurysm. Unfortunately, the patient died of sepsis following surgery. Undaunted by this complication, Cooper performed his first successful ligation of the carotid artery in 1808 on another patient with a cervical carotid aneurysm. The patient suffered no untoward effects from the ligation and lived until 1821 (3).

In the 19th century, a number of carotid ligations were performed by various surgeons for the treatment of various diseases such as cervical carotid aneurysms and other vascular malformations. Benjamin Travers reported a case of carotid ligation in a patient who presented with carotid-cavernous sinus fistula in 1809 (1). In 1868, Pilz published a series of 600 cases of carotid ligation for hemorrhage or cervical aneurysm with an overall mortality of 43% (1).

Carrea et al. reported the first successful carotid reconstruction procedure in Buenos Aires in 1951 (4). The patient presented with symptoms of a stroke, and arteriography demonstrated a stenosis of the internal carotid artery (ICA). Carrea performed a direct anastomosis of the external carotid artery (ECA) to the distal ICA following resection of the stenotic segment.

The surgical technique of thromboendarterectomy was first introduced to the United States by Wylie in 1951 (5). He documented use of this technique for the removal of atherosclerotic plaques in the aortoiliac segments. The success of this procedure on the large vessels of the abdomen and lower extremities set the stage for the application of this technique to the cervical carotid vessels.

DeBakey performed the first successful carotid endarterectomy (CEA) in 1953 (6). The patient presented with symptoms of a frank stroke. Angiogram confirmed the presence of a total occlusion of the left ICA. Postoperatively, arteriography confirmed the presence of flow in the ICA (7).

Carotid reconstruction for the treatment of carotid occlusive diseases and transient ischemic attacks (TIAs) was presented by Eastcott et al. in 1954 (8). They reported the case of a 66-year-old woman who presented with episodes of TIAs that had been getting progressively worse. Angiography demonstrated the presence of near occlusion of the left ICA. She underwent direct anastomosis of the common carotid artery (CCA) to the ICA following resection of the diseased portion of the ICA. She tolerated the procedure quite well and suffered no further attacks of ischemia or infarction related to the left ICA. This case represented the beginning of the exploration of carotid artery reconstruction as a primary treatment for the carotid occlusive diseases. It is a source of great satisfaction to neurovascular surgeons that at the present time this elegant and enjoyable operation, nearly 40-years-old, has now been unequivocally shown to prevent stroke in well-chosen patients with clear and unambiguous clinical findings.

SCIENTIFIC FOUNDATION FOR CAROTID ARTERY RECONSTRUCTION

Diseases of the carotid circulatory system can be divided into asymptomatic (always and still the subject of great debate) and symptomatic forms. Patients with asymptomatic carotid diseases include those with asymptomatic carotid bruits, symptoms referable to one carotid territory with radiographic demonstration of clinically silent contralateral carotid stenosis or ulceration, and those who are found to have auscultatory or radiographic evidence of carotid pathology while being prepared for their major surgical procedures (most commonly coronary or peripheral vascular surgery). Symptomatic carotid disease encompasses a spectrum of presentations from TIAs to stroke in evolution and completed stroke, and includes acute or subacute carotid occlusion as well as the so-called "stump syndromes." In the last decade, several domestic and international government funded multicenter randomized cooperative trials have changed the practice of carotid reconstruction for both asymptomatic and symptomatic patients. Clearly, the scientific rationale for carotid artery reconstruction differs from the principles outlined in the first edition of this book (9), and we should carefully analyze the class 1 evidence trial data for both types of clinical presentation.

Asymptomatic Carotid Disease

Asymptomatic Bruit

Surgery for asymptomatic carotid disease has long been controversial. At the time of the first edition of this book, no level 1 evidence was in place to justify asymptomatic carotid reconstruction. The results of the Asymptomatic Carotid Atherosclerosis Study (ACAS) and Asymptomatic Carotid Surgery Trials (ACST) (10,11) have changed many opinions and have validated the practice of CEA for asymptomatic disease in selected cases. It seems unlikely that trials such as ACAS/ACST will ever be repeated, considering the definitive results of the study; consequently, in my practice we have tailored surgical recommendations to comply with ACAS findings, and we have devised strategies to deal with and address the questions (such as the status of women) that ACAS did not answer. Let us first examine the data on which we based clinical decisions prior to ACAS, and then re-evaluate that data in the light of the ACAS/ACST evidence.

Carotid bruits are heard in 3% to 4% of the asymptomatic U.S. population over 45 years of age and are present in 10% to 23% of patients in referral populations with symptomatic atherosclerosis in other arterial distributions. Many major studies advocated surgery for asymptomatic carotid bruits (12,13). These two referenced studies followed a group of unoperated patients with asymptomatic bruits and reported higher rates of neurologic sequelae (with stroke rates of 15–17%) as compared to operated controls. Neither report, however, documented the relationship of the neurologic events to the territory of the carotid bruit (e.g., ipsilateral or contralateral), nor was it reported which of the patients suffering acute cerebrovascular accident (CVA) had experienced a warning TIA prior to that event (which would have justified prophylactic endarterectomy in most centers). These questions have been addressed, however, in several subsequent population studies (14,15). The first study reported on a series of 72 patients with carotid bruits, 10 of whom went on to develop strokes, but in whom the strokes occurred mostly in different vascular territories (14). In the second report, data from the Framingham study confirmed that asymptomatic bruit predicted an increased risk of neurologic events, but that the majority of these events were either in other cerebrovascular territories or were etiologically related to noncarotid factors, e.g., aneurysms, lacunar infarcts, or emboli following myocardial infarction (MI) (15). Both studies confirmed that patients with asymptomatic bruit are at increased risk for cerebrovascular and/or cardiac problems, but could not provide justification for prophylactic surgery for the asmyptomatic bruit alone.

There was some evidence to suggest that silent, small cerebral infarction [seen on computed tomography (CT)] may justify CEA in otherwise asymptomatic patients. Norris and Zhu (16) reported a significantly higher incidence of silent infarcts ipsilateral to high-grade (>75%) carotid stenosis compared to lower grades. Based on this evidence, we considered (and still do) lacunes of this type combined with severe stenosis to be a relative indication for prophylactic carotid reconstruction.

The question of surgery for critical high-grade asymptomatic stenosis remained open and was the subject of considerable debate among vascular surgeons, neurosurgeons, and neurologists. Hemodynamic studies suggested that critical reductions in cerebral blood flow may not be reached until 75% to 84% diameter stenosis has occurred, indicating that stenosis must be of a very high grade to be significant (17). One group, using prospective noninvasive studies, showed a higher propensity for neurologic events or acute carotid occlusion in lesions found to be 80% or more stenotic (18), and another documented the protective effect of surgery in these patients (19). On the basis of these reports, many surgeons felt justified in correcting such severe but otherwise asymptomatic lesions. Chambers and Norris, on the other hand, reported that in asymptomatic patients with stenosis of all degrees, the risk of cardiac ischemia was higher than that of stroke. In their series, although the risk of cerebral ischemic events was highest in patients with severe carotid artery stenosis, in most instances these patients did not have strokes without some sort of warning event (20). More recently, Norris et al. (21) followed 696 patients for a mean of 41 months with noninvasive studies. While the combined TIA/stroke rate for patients with >75% stenosis was a significant 10.5%, the ipsilateral stroke rate (without warning TIA) was 2.5% for patients with >75% stenosis, and 1.1% with <75% stenosis. These data reemphasized the need for surgical action in symptomatic high-grade stenosis patients, but did not identify a high-risk asymptomatic subgroup (21). Many reviews on this subject recommended medical management of the patient with asymptomatic carotid bruit or stenosis with antiplatelet aggregating therapy (ASA) and attention to contributing risk factors (hypertension), with surgical intervention deferred until such time as frank TIAs develop (22–25).

The continuing controversy over asymptomatic carotid disease spawned several large clinical trials. Prospective, randomized trials comparing medical and surgical therapies in patients with asymptomatic ICA stenosis include the Carotid Artery Stenosis with Asymptomatic Narrowing Operation Versus Aspirin (CASANOVA) study, the Mayo Asymptomatic Carotid Endarterectomy Trial (MACE), the Veterans Administration Cooperative Trial on Asymptomatic Carotid Stenosis (VAAST), and the ACAS. Three of these four trials were negative for a surgical benefit in stroke prevention, but the fourth trial (ACAS) was positive and authoritative, and no further North American trials are planned or likely to be done. The largest, and most recent asymptomatic carotid surgery randomized trial— the ACST— trial was just completed in the United Kingdom and Europe (26). Gratifyingly, this trial also supports asymptomatic carotid reconstruction, just as the ACAS did (11).

The CASANOVA study randomized patients from the general population to immediate surgery versus antiplatelet therapy alone and best medical management. The stenosis criterion was 50% to 90% by noninvasive testing or angiography. Both arms received best medical management including aspirin (1000 mg/d) and dipyridamole (225 mg/d). The follow-up was three years and the study size was 410 patients. Endpoints were death and stroke. Two-hundred-and-six patients were randomized to immediate surgery and 204 patients were randomized to antiplatelet therapy alone. One-hundred-and-eighteen of the 204 patients in the nonsurgical arm had delayed endarterectomy during the follow-up period secondary to TIA, progressive severe stenosis (>90%), bilateral stenosis (>50%), or contralateral stenosis (>50%). The study found no statistically significant difference in outcome between the surgical and nonsurgical arms (10.7% and 11.3%, respectively). The unusual study design of CASANOVA limits its statistical validity (27). By its very design, excluding high-risk patients from the medical arm and allowing crossovers, the CASANOVA trial was biased against surgery from the onset.

The MACE study enrolled 71 patients with >50% stenosis by noninvasive testing. The planned follow-up was two years. The nonsurgical arm received best medical management and aspirin (80 mg/d). The surgical arm did not receive aspirin. Only Mayo Clinic patients were randomized to the treatment arms. The study was terminated prematurely because of increased frequency of MI in surgical arm patients (who did not receive aspirin). At termination, too few patients were enrolled to assess statistical significance. The major finding of MACE was that aspirin was appropriate for the peri-operative and postoperative period unless contraindicated (28).

The Veterans Administration Asymptomatic Stenosis Trial (VAAST) enrolled only men from VA centers and randomized them to surgical and nonsurgical arms, both of which received best medical management and aspirin (1300 mg/d). The stenosis criterion for entry and randomization was >50% by angiography. The follow-up was five years and the study population was 444 patients (211/444 surgical and 233/444 non surgical). Participating centers were screened and required to demonstrate a perioperative morbidity and mortality of <3%. At four year follow-up, the combined incidence of ipsilateral TIA or stroke was 8% and 20.6% for the surgical and nonsurgical arms, respectively ($p < 0.001$). The sample size was not large enough to show statistical significance for stroke alone; the recommendation was that surgery was effective in preventing subsequent TIAs in asymptomatic patients (29).

The second largest of the asymptomatic trials was the ACAS. The trialists randomized 1659 patients (834 treated medically and 825 patients treated surgically) between ages 40 and 79 years with 60% to 99% ICA stenosis to 325 mg of aspirin plus risk-factor management or endarterectomy plus medical therapy. The trial was stopped prematurely because of a demonstrated benefit for surgery in all patients with >60% linear stenosis. (It would be considered unethical to continue randomization of patients in the face of a known surgical benefit.) After median follow-up of 2.7 years, the aggregate estimated risk over five years for ipsilateral stroke or perioperative stroke or death was 5.1% for patients who underwent surgery and 11% for patients treated medically. CEA reduced the estimated five-year risk for ipsilateral stroke by 1% per year. The benefit did not extend to major stroke alone and could not be demonstrated in women as a subgroup, probably because of the small numbers and premature closure of the trial. [There was also a higher perioperative complication rate for women in ACAS; two later studies, however, have shown that no true gender-related risk exists (30,31).] The success of the ACAS trial, and of the operative procedure, depended on maintenance of a perioperative morbidity and mortality of less than 3% (10).

Finally, ACST randomized 3120 patients during 1993–2003 to either CEA or indefinite deferral (medical management). The perioperative 30-day stroke/death rate was 3.1%. Five-year stroke risk in the CEA group was 3.8% and in the medical group 11%, a statistically significant benefit for surgery. Unlike ACAS, benefit was shown independently for both males and females. The trialists recommended CEA for all patients <75-years-old with 70% or greater ultrasound confirmed carotid stenosis, with the conviction that surgery halved the risk of subsequent stroke, even after perioperative stroke/death rate was factored in (11).

We can say with confidence that the indications for surgical reconstruction in asymptomatic patients have been confirmed by level 1 clinical trials evidence since the first edition of this book went to press. My surgical policy follows directly from the ACAS/ACST guidelines. I offer surgery to patients with a five-year life expectancy who have 60% or greater stenosis, including women. For women I explain the details of the data and the weaker evidence that a protective benefit may apply to them as a subgroup. Most patients, in my experience, choose surgery when informed and educated in this way. The latest iteration of the American Heart Association (AHA) Guidelines for CEA confirms this surgical approach for patients with surgical risk <3% and a five-year life expectancy (32).

Contralateral Carotid Stenosis

A number of clinical studies, primarily retrospective, were undertaken with the goal of ascertaining the risks of long-term neurologic sequelae in patients with contralateral carotid stenosis managed nonoperatively. The critical point, much as in the follow-up of asymptomatic bruits, was to determine what percentage of these patients progressed to frank stroke in the appropriate carotid distribution without warning TIAs. Most of the studies specified 50% stenosis of the contralateral carotid as the criterion for significant disease (33–37). In three of these reports, no patients followed up for contralateral asymptomatic lesions developed a stroke without warning TIAs (35–37). In two other reports, a few patients did develop such strokes, but the incidence was invariably less than 3%, and thus less than the accepted risks of surgical morbidity and mortality (33, 34). A single study included all patients with contralateral stenosis from 1% to 99% and reported the incidence of direct stroke in unoperated patients to be 3%; these authors recommended prophylactic surgery on this basis, and also concluded that the percent stenosis did not correlate with the risk of neurological sequelae (38). Aside from this group's findings, however, no authors could demonstrate that prophylactic surgery for contralateral lesions of greater than 50% stenosis had any protective effect in the absence of clinical symptoms referable to that lesion.

The question of progression to 80% or greater on the contralateral side was specifically addressed by Roederer et al. (19). In noninvasive follow-up, they found that the rate of neurologic events significantly increased once an 80% lesion developed. They argued that these asymptomatic stenoses of >80% should be reconstructed. Their data seem prescient now in view of the ACAS and ACST results discussed above, and it is our policy to recommend surgical reconstruction for contralateral silent stenosis opposite either an asymptomatic or symptomatic lesion, assuming that baseline ACAS/ACST criteria are satisfied.

Carotid Risks in Noncarotid Preoperative Patients

Randomized cooperative trial data (class 1 evidence) is definitive, and clearly has sufficient power to change surgical practice. It should be clear by now that the ACAS/ACST trials superseded a substantial number of smaller clinical series, many of which could not demonstrate a surgical benefit. One such clinical issue that was extensively studied was the proper management of preoperative patients who are found to have auscultatory or radiographic evidence of otherwise silent carotid artery disease. A number of studies addressed this problem. One early group performed prophylactic endarterectomies in 34 surgical patients and was able to demonstrate low morbidity and good long-term survival following the procedure (39). It was not clear, however, that their patients were at increased risk for cerebrovascular events, and thus whether these prophylactic procedures, albeit safe in their hands, were necessary. This point was addressed further by a series of retrospective studies of surgical patients identified to have asymptomatic bruits but followed without carotid surgery (40–43). These studies established the incidence of asymptomatic bruits in random preoperative patients to be near 15%. Although they documented a perioperative stroke rate of about 1% in their patient groups, none of these investigators could find a correlation between presence or location of carotid bruits and risk of perioperative stroke. Further investigations (44–47) prospectively examined asymptomatic bruit patients with noninvasive carotid studies in an attempt to correlate percent stenosis with risk of perioperative stroke. Although some of their reports documented higher perioperative mortality in the carotid stenosis groups (44,45), these deaths were primarily attributable to an increased risk of MI, and once again no correlation could be demonstrated between bruit or stenosis and perioperative stroke risk. In one prospective study of preoperative patients with asymptomatic bruits only, 14% incidence of bruits in this group was confirmed, and all strokes (0.7% of patients) were found in patients having coronary bypass surgery (48). The concept that the increased risk of perioperative stroke in coronary bypass patients arises from femoral arterial cannulation rather than incidental carotid disease with carotid embolization and/or hypoperfusion was supported by a Canadian study that found femoral cannulation to be the only statistically significant common denominator among a group of bypass patients with embolic stroke (49). Furlan (50) studied patients undergoing coronary artery bypass graft (CABG) who had angiographically documented asymptomatic stenosis greater than 50% and showed that stroke risk was not increased in patients with either <90% stenosis or with total ICA occlusion. There was an insufficient number of patients in the 90% -to- 99% group to allow statistical conclusions.

While ACAS/ACST validate carotid reconstruction for asymptomatic stenosis, the timing issue vis-a-vis other planned surgery is not as clear. Our previous policy of "watchful waiting" for patients with silent stenosis undergoing other surgical procedures is no longer appropriate, and we reconstruct silent carotid disease when it is identified in patients scheduled for noncarotid surgery. Whether a staged or a reverse-staged operative strategy is best has not been answered, and remains the judgment of the individual surgeon taking all patient factors into account.

Hollenhorst Plaque

In 1961, Hollenhorst described 31 patients with orange-yellow or copper colored plaques observed ophthalmoscopically at bifurcations of the retinal arterioles. Twenty-seven of these patients had occlusive disease in the carotid tree and four in the vertebral basilar tree. He also described five patients who underwent CEA and subsequently were found to have showers of these plaques in the retina postoperatively. Hollenhorst felt that these plaques represented cholesterol emboli from the extracranial circulation and that their presence warranted aggressive investigation of the cardiovascular and cerebrovascular system for surgically correctable disease (51). The atheromatous nature of this embolic material was confirmed by David's pathologic report in 1963 (52).

It is important to distinguish symptomatic retinal plaques from asymptomatic ones. Multiple authors have reported plaques associated with either amaurosis fugax or retinal artery occlusion with visual field deficits and there is little doubt that these represent symptomatic carotid lesions (53–55). Russell classifies these refractile cholesterol-containing flakes as his third type of retinal emboli, and points out that they customarily disappear from the retina within a few weeks, with or without leaving a permanent field deficit. Once again these symptomatic lesions certainly deserve active investigation for carotid origin embolization.

In 1973, Hollenhorst's group reported on 208 consecutive patients observed to have retinal cholesterol emboli who had been followed up for at least six years. This group was mixed and many of them had visual symptoms associated with their cholesterol emboli. This group of patients had significantly decreased survival compared to a heterogeneous comparison group with a survival rate 13% less than expected in the first year increasing to 80% less than expected by the eighth year of observation. The cause of death in many of these patients was related to diffuse vascular disease with MI being the greatest factor. Hollenhorst concluded on the basis of these data that these plaques warrant aggressive cardiac and cerebrovascular investigation (56).

Patients with truly asymptomatic retinal cholesterol emboli represent a much more unusual and smaller group. Very little data are available as to the natural history and prognosis of these patients. Bruno et al. (57) recently studied 70 consecutive men with asymptomatic retinal cholesterol emboli and compared them to a control group of 21 randomly selected subjects without retinal emboli. Patients in their study group had a significantly higher prevalence of hypertension and smoking history than did the control group. The prevalence of carotid stenosis ≥50% ipsilateral to the embolus was only 13%, however, and this was not significantly different from that in control subjects. However, carotid stenosis ≥50% on either side was more common in patients with asymptomatic retinal cholesterol emboli. According to Bruno's data, asymptomatic retinal cholesterol emboli do indicate a higher prevalence of systemic vascular disease and of ischemic heart disease, similar to that reported by Pfaffenbach and Hollenhorst (56). Their data, however, do not support the concept that asymptomatic retinal cholesterol emboli are the harbingers of cerebrovascular events or of the presence of an unstable carotid atherosclerotic plaque. In keeping with this, it should be noted that asymptomatic retinal cholesterol emboli were not considered entry criteria for the North American Symptomatic Carotid Endarterectomy Trial (NASCET).

What then can be said about the presence of Hollenhorst plaques? Certainly, any identifiable retinal lesion with visual symptoms must be considered a symptomatic carotid event until proven otherwise and warrants full investigation. I have performed CEA on many patients whose initial presentation was visual loss from central retinal artery occlusion. The significance of asymptomatic lesions in the retina is more obscure and not as extensively studied. Available small series data imply that these patients do not represent a high-risk group. Notwithstanding, it has been my inclination to actively investigate these patients on the few occasions when absolutely no visual symptoms can be elicited and I have been aggressive in the management of these lesions, consistent with my standard approach to asymptomatic disease. I am pleased that ACST and ACAS data support this, and validate carotid reconstruction in such patients when an appropriate degree of stenosis is confirmed.

Symptomatic Carotid Disease

Symptomatic disease in the carotid circulation encompasses a spectrum of presentations from classical carotid TIAs to frank embolic or thrombotic stroke. It is at times paradoxical, in that the degree of collateral circulation may allow severe carotid pathology to present with only minimal symptomatology (e.g., there is a finite incidence of carotid occlusion presenting with TIAs alone). Whereas the discussion of asymptomatic carotid disease involved primarily a comparison of operated patients versus unoperated control groups, any consideration of surgery for symptomatic carotid disease must be based on objective comparison of surgical morbidity and results of both the natural history of the disease process and the best available medical therapy. The surgical risk in elective CEAs performed in major centers approaches 3%, as previously mentioned, and this figure should be used for evaluation of therapeutic choices. Guidelines for acceptable surgical morbidity and mortality have been published by both the AHA Stroke Council (58) and the American College of Physicians (59). Evidence-based guidelines for asymptomatic and symptomatic carotid reconstruction have been elegantly revised by an AHA working group, and should be considered definitive (32).

Transient Ischemic Attacks

Three well-accepted studies have documented that the risk of stroke following a first classical carotid TIA approximates 5% per year (60–62). Equally important are data showing that 51% of all such strokes occur in the first year following initial TIA and that 21% occur in the first month following such an event (63). It is only after the first six months that the risk of stroke falls to, and remains, 5% annually. This malignant natural history has prompted approaches to medical therapy. Anticoagulation has proven difficult to control in an outpatient population. Such therapy has also been shown to be associated with a high risk of intracranial hemorrhage which, in one series of patients aged 55 to 74, was eight times greater than in a control group (64). Furthermore, all studies of anticoagulant therapy in TIAs failed to demonstrate differences in mortality between treated and untreated groups. The consequent decline in use of anticoagulation as primary therapy for TIAs was paralleled by a great interest in antiplatelet-aggregating agents. In the American controlled study of aspirin therapy for cerebral ischemia (65), antiplatelet-aggregating therapy was shown to decrease the incidence of recurrent TIAs but did not significantly decrease the long-term incidence of stroke in treated patients. The Canadian study of aspirin and sulfinpyrazone, however, did show a significant

31% decrease in long-term risk of stroke or death (66). This risk reduction was sex dependent, and in males a 48% risk reduction was demonstrated. Dipyridamole has not supplemented aspirin's effect on risk reduction of stroke after TIA (67). Assuming a 5% annual risk of stroke in untreated patients then, the best medical therapy presently available reduces this risk by nearly one half, to 2½% per year.

Much like asymptomatic carotid disease, symptomatic carotid disease became the focus of several randomized cooperative trials in the late 1980s. An European Carotid Surgery Trial (ECST) of symptomatic patients in all subgroups from 0% to 99% stenosis was paralleled by two trials in North America, the NASCET and the VA Cooperative Trial of Symptomatic Carotid Disease (VASST). On February 22, 1991, the entry of patients with greater than 70% stenosis into the NASCET trial was stopped because an endpoint was reached in which it was clearly demonstrated that surgical treatment of these patients was superior to medical management (68,69). The NASCET trial continued entry and follow-up of patients from 30% to 69% stenosis who were clinically symptomatic. Later analysis of the NASCET data showed a surgical benefit, albeit more modest, for patients with angiographic stenosis of 50% or more (70).

Concurrent with release of data from the NASCET trial, a similar release by the European group (coincidentally during the same week) reported that a clear surgical benefit was found in patients with 70% to 99% stenosis in that trial as well (71). At the same time these investigators declared that medical therapy was clearly superior for symptomatic patients with stenosis less than 30% (a group not studied by NASCET). The European trial also continued to enter patients with between 30% to 70% stenosis; paradoxically, they were not ultimately able to demonstrate a surgical benefit in the moderate stenosis group (72). This contradiction can be explained and reconciled by the more rigorous angiographic measurement system employed in the NASCET; many "high-grade" stenosis ECST patients were considered only "moderate grade" when measured with the NASCET system (where N is the linear diameter at the area of greatest narrowing, and D is the greatest diameter of the normal artery distal to the carotid bulb.

$$\text{Percent (\%) stenosis} = (1 - N/D) \times 100$$

and moderate-grade ECST patients (in whom a surgical benefit was not demonstrated) fall below the 50% NASCET criterion. When imaging data were later normalized so that the NASCET and ECST groups could be directly compared, ECST also showed a modest benefit for surgery in 50% to 69% stenosis patients (73).

The VASST was terminated early secondary to preliminary results from the two aforementioned trials. Though 5000 patients were screened at 16 participating VA centers, only 193 men were randomized to best medical management (98 men) and surgical (91 men) treatment arms (74). Angiography was performed on all patients and greater than two-thirds of the population had >70% stenosis. There was a mean follow-up of 11.9 months. The risk of stroke or crescendo TIA was 7.7% versus 19.4% (surgical vs. nonsurgical, $p = 0.028$). There was a significant surgical benefit in patients with >70% stenosis. Sample size at 50% to 69% stenosis was too small to draw any statistically significant conclusions. Surgical benefit was appreciated as soon as two months status postrandomization and was maintained throughout follow-up. Total perioperative risk was 5.5% (perioperative morbidity of 2.2% plus perioperative mortality of 3.3%).

The exciting data from the NASCET, European, and VASST trials showed that surgical treatment is the best option in patients with classical carotid TIAs and greater than 50% stenosis demonstrated by arteriography.

Acute Neurological Deficit

Surgical intervention via CEA is often not a consideration in cases of acute stroke, for several reasons. First, many patients presenting with acute neurologic deficits have as their primary problem a noncarotid event such as hypertensive hemorrhage or cardiogenic emboli. Second, even those patients identified to have carotid embolic disease as the cause of their neurologic deterioration have fared poorly when subjected to emergency carotid surgery. In one early study, more than 50% of such patients suffered a fatal intracranial hemorrhage within 72 hours of emergency endarterectomy (75). Other investigators have reported moderate success, however, with emergency surgery in patients fulfilling strict preoperative criteria. These criteria include crescendo TIAs (attacks abruptly increasing in frequency to at least several per day) in patients with severe stenosis; stroke following angiography; stroke following endarterectomy if thrombosis is present; and disappearance of a previously auscultated bruit in patients awaiting elective carotid surgery (presumably indicating acute occlusion) (76–79). Subsequently, encouraging results were reported by two groups performing emergency surgery for crescendo TIAs and stroke in evolution clinically and radiographically localized to one carotid artery (79,80). Goldstone and Moore (79) emphasized, however, that patients with depressed levels of consciousness or acute fixed deficits were excluded from their surgical series, and agree with other authors that such findings must be taken as absolute contraindications for emergency CEA.

The retrospective series of Walters et al. (81) from the Massachusetts General Hospital confirmed many of these conclusions. In their 64 patients (a mixed series including 16 total occlusions), clinical results were best in patients with mild to moderate deficit and a rapid course from onset of deficit to surgery. Like previous authors, they recommended surgery for patients who had loss of bruit or deficit following angiography and/or endarterectomy. They also recommended emergency surgery for crescendo TIAs in patients with angiographic severe stenosis and distal flow delay, ICA stenosis with intraluminal filling defect, or demonstrated acute complete occlusion (81).

A study of acute carotid occlusion and profound neurologic deficit was reported by Meyer et al. (82) in a series of 34 patients with complete occlusion who had emergency CEA. All patients had profound neurologic deficit including hemiplegia and aphasia. Patency was restored in 94% of cases and they documented nine patients (26.5%) with normal postoperative neurological function, four patients (11.8%) with minimal neurological deficit, 10 (29.4%) with moderate hemiparesis but improved from preoperative level, four (11.8%) with unchanged hemiplegia, and seven (20.6%) dead. The authors of this study felt that these results compared favorably with the natural history of complete acute carotid occlusion with profound deficit and suggested that the presence of favorable collateral circulation on angiography was a positive prognostic sign for neurologic recovery (82).

At present, then, emergency CEA is indicated only in a specific subpopulation of stroke patients, that is, those with documented carotid etiology for a progressive but nondebilitating ischemic event, or those in whom evidence of acute thrombosis is present and who can be operated upon within several hours of the event (18).

It should be mentioned that a fine line of distinction is drawn between emergency and urgent carotid artery surgery. The data from the NASCET study clearly show that surgery is the best treatment for symptomatic patients with ipsilateral stenosis greater than 50% (69,70). When such patients, particularly those with high-grade or preocclusive stenosis, are identified in my practice, and they are neurologically stable, we consider them urgent cases, and perform surgery as soon as possible, customarily the day after angiography. Almost all of these patients are managed with systemic heparin anticoagulation, which is continued up to and throughout the surgical procedure (as discussed later). Tretter et al. (83) have elegantly analyzed their risk factors in a large Cleveland Clinic series of "nonelective" CEA; the demonstrated increased risk is attributable to cardiopulmonary risk factors rather than neurologic events.

There are new data addressing the combination of intravenous thrombolysis for stroke (tPA) and urgent carotid reconstruction. McPherson et al. (84) operated within 48 hours of tPA administration on five patients without complications when a high-grade residual stenosis was identified, demonstrating feasibility and safety with this approach. Eckstein reports a mixed series of 14 patients with either cervical ICA or intracerebral major vessel occlusions (MCA, ACA) or both, who received either staged tPA followed by CEA (3 cases), or in 11 cases emergency CEA with concurrent intraoperative angiographic selective urokinase injection intracranially (85). In these patients, all of whom had a severe preoperative neurological deficit, four made a complete recovery and six more had only minor residual strokes. This is a complex strategy, but it does indicate that aggressive and individually tailored approaches to stroke, which infold CEA as a treatment arm, are appropriate.

Complete Carotid Occlusion

Complete carotid occlusion, like many of the carotid syndromes, may present without symptoms, with TIAs or fluctuating neurologic deficit, or with frank stroke. Some overlap exists, therefore, in the literature dealing with complete occlusion and in that addressing emergency endarterectomy for stroke. Aside from the acute nondebilitating neurologic deficits previously discussed, surgery for subacute carotid occlusion has been performed both to restore blood flow to the ipsilateral hemisphere and to prevent emboli originating from the stump of an occluded ICA from propagating distally. The ability to reestablish flow in such situations is dependent upon the duration of the occlusion, with several authors reporting 100% success in reopening these arteries within 7 days (86,87). Delayed surgery has been less promising (87,88), and successful restoration of flow in late surgical cases (5 weeks) appears to be dependent upon the degree of collateral filling present from intracavernous and intrapetrous carotid branches (86,89). One study has documented 58% patency at six months by follow-up angiography (90), while a more recent study by McCormick et al. (91) reported 88% wide patency and only one reocclusion at a mean 28 months follow-up. In one recent series of surgery for documented acute ICA occlusion, patency was established in 83% of cases and 74% of patients had neurological improvement at three to six months (92). In another series, Paty et al. (93) were able to open 30% of carotids explored within two weeks; in the rest an ECA endarterectomy was combined with ICA stump ligation.

Surgical intervention for complete carotid occlusion appears indicated in an extremely limited group of patients who present with either acute nondebilitating deficit directly attributable to such occlusions, or with ischemic symptoms referable to embolization from an occluded stump. In these highly selected cases, thrombo-endarterectomy carries a low surgical risk and, depending on the duration of occlusion and degree of collateral filling, has a reasonable chance of achieving long-term patency.

Stump Syndromes

As mentioned previously, in recent years attention has focused on the importance of the often-found "stump" of an occluded ICA as a possible source for ipsilateral embolic phenomena (94,95). The presumed mechanism for these TIAs is through embolization of debris from the stump through external carotid–ophthalmic artery collaterals. This mechanism has been documented angiographically (95,96). Obviously, before the carotid stump can be implicated as the etiologic source, the presence of major collaterals and the absence of other significant atheromatous disease must be documented with four-vessel angiography. In cases where this etiology seems clear, however, and where reopening of the internal carotid cannot be achieved, I surgically ligate and oversew (from the inside out) the offending stump, with concurrent open endarterectomy of the CCA and ECA, and, for the past several years, placement of a common to external roof patch Hemashield angioplasty (97). (See Section 5-2 for details.) I monitor these patients with the same EEG criteria as an internal CEA, and am prepared to shunt the external carotid if changes are noted. In my experience, by using strict selection criteria, this procedure has been an effective therapy for recurrent neurologic phenomena, and has the added benefit that an occasional stump exploration may lead to backbleeding and the reestablishment of anterograde internal carotid flow. I feel strongly that treatment of such stumps in appropriate patients is as important for stroke prevention as is treatment of any other symptomatic carotid lesion.

Special Considerations with Recent Stroke

Finally, it should be noted that a number of authors who customarily advocate selective shunting have found intraoperative monitoring to be unreliable in patients who have had recent reversible ischemic neurologic deficit (RIND) or stroke. These groups recommend empirical shunt placement in all such cases (98,99). Likewise, although many cerebrovascular surgeons empirically recommend a three to six weeks delay prior to performing CEA in patients with fresh but nondebilitating strokes, especially those with CT or magnetic resonance imaging (MRI) findings of large infarct and mass effect (and thus with presumed defective autoregulation), three later studies have shown that patients who are neurologically stable probably are at no greater surgical risk in the early poststroke period than TIA patients, and that the high-risk subgroup is that of patients who remain neurologically unstable at the time of surgery (100–102).

Clinical Evaluation

Patients present to the cerebrovascular surgeon in many different ways. Asymptomatic patients are customarily elective and seen in the office or clinic. Patients with TIAs may present likewise or may be seen as hospital consults. Patients with crescendo TIAs, frank stroke, and/or acute occlusion will no doubt be seen as emergencies while in hospital. The latter patients may or may not be heparinized and may be in various states of neurologic deterioration.

Elective patients undergo a rapid workup with the goal of performing surgery as soon as possible. I continue to prefer formal angiography in most cases including arch and selective injection of both common carotids. Attention to intracranial cross filling is also useful in assessing collateral patterns and I request biplane cervical angiography in order to determine the anatomical relationship of the ECAs and ICAs. It is helpful to have bony landmarks imaged on the lateral angiographic films to ascertain the height of the carotid bulb in relation to the cervical spine, the angle of the mandible, and the hyoid bone. Although I use duplex scanning as a screening procedure and for postoperative follow-up, I do not believe it is routinely needed if patients have already undergone magnetic resonance angiography (MRA) or angiography.

A topic of current interest is that of operating on patients based on MRA or CT angiography alone (103,104). This has become a common practice among neurovascular surgeons seeking to avoid the small but finite risk of angiography, nearly 1% in ACAS (10). Many surgeons have accepted MRA alone for surgical decision making and planning, although there is to my mind no question that the anatomical detail is not as rich. I do not operate on patients on the basis of duplex scanning alone. There is compelling evidence to suggest that noninvasive studies alone are inferior for surgical decision making if low-risk angiography is available (105).

Patients who are seen for potential carotid surgery are customarily on aspirin or some form of anticoagulation; if they are not, they are started on aspirin at the time of first visit. I do not stop preoperative aspirin therapy in preparation for surgery, but I do discontinue ticlopidine or clopidrogel at least one week preoperation. Likewise in patients who are heparinized for crescendo TIAs, I customarily maintain full anticoagulation up to, and throughout, the surgical procedure. In such patients, we check the activated clotting times (ACT) value in the operating room at the beginning of the case; most often the anticoagulation is too low despite continuous heparin and a small bolus must be given. As mentioned, I have no hesitation to operate on fully heparinized patients, and in special cases (bilateral crescendo TIAs, mechanical heart valves), I have maintained full heparinization postoperatively then converted to warfarin without any gap; the risk of this is postoperative wound hematoma, and in my series I have encountered two of these (see Fig. 4-4), both in patients with mechanical valves treated with constant anticoagulation therapy.

The remainder of the preoperative evaluation is standard. A careful neurologic examination is performed and a history is carefully obtained for stereotypic TIAs in any carotid distribution. A history of cardiac disease warrants cardiology consultation and patients who smoke are advised to quit as far in advance of the surgical procedure as possible.

Special Surgical Considerations

Several special situations in carotid patients were previously considered relative contraindications to successful reconstruction but these have become more acceptable with recent advances in radiologic, surgical, and anesthetic techniques.

Plaque Ulceration

The correlation of plaque ulceration with ischemic neurologic symptoms and need for surgery is difficult for several reasons. First, studies have shown interobserver variability either on ultrasound or arteriographic examinations, and poor correlation between pathologic specimens and radiographically demonstrated ulceration. Second, in symptomatic patients, deep ulceration is most commonly found in conjunction with significant degrees of carotid stenosis, and it becomes difficult to separate clinical symptomatology between these two findings (106,107). The most recent data from the NASCET study, however, shows that in medically treated patients with 70% to 99% stenosis (now proven to be unequivocal surgical candidates), the presence of plaque ulceration in conjunction with stenosis significantly increases the risk of stroke (108).

The significance of intraplaque hemorrhage as a predictor of ischemic symptoms is unclear. Although Gomez (106) suggested that intraplaque hemorrhage was found much more commonly in patients with symptomatic carotid disease, other studies suggest that there is a low correlation between ischemic symptoms and plaque hematoma in CEA patients (109).

Critical Stenosis

The question of critical stenosis has recently been well addressed. Critical stenosis need no longer be debated. Surgery is appropriate and proven by class 1 evidence for 50% or greater symptomatic lesions and for 60% or greater asymptomatic lesions. In light of these data, "critical" stenosis now only indicates a need for expeditious surgery and in many cases for preoperative systemic anticoagulation.

Intraluminal Thrombus

The problem of surgical timing in patients with angiographically demonstrated propagating intraluminal thrombus remains an open question among cerebrovascular experts. There are two types of thrombus seen on imaging studies: the small "bullet type"—localized to the area of critical stenosis, and the longer "propagating type"—extending far up the internal carotid, sometimes into the supraclinoid region (see Fig. 2-18). For the bullet type, which can be easily controlled by cross-clamping above the thrombus at open surgery, we do not hesitate to proceed. The best management for the propagating type is less clear. Several authors have documented that an increased risk of perioperative or intraoperative stroke must be accepted when operating on patients who have propagating clot that may extend beyond the area of internal carotid cross-clamping or that is more friable and prone to dislodgment than the usual carotid plaque (110–112). Review of the literature suggests that a period of observation with full heparinization prior to undertaking surgical therapy may reduce the morbidity and mortality in these patients (110,112,113). Clearly, the choice of therapy must be tailored for individual cases. It is equally clear, however, that intraluminal thrombus is a therapeutic emergency but not necessarily a surgical emergency, rather the identification of propagating thrombus should provoke a careful and measured response to the situation. As one author has suggested, heparinization should probably be instituted in every case followed by consideration of endarterectomy in patients who are neurologically stable, and by a delayed surgical plan following a period of expectant observation in neurologically unstable patients or those with serious intercurrent illness or hypercoagulable state (113). In patients who present with TIAs (which in my experience have always resolved with anticoagulation) and an intraluminal thrombus, I have opted for delayed surgery (at six weeks, following repeat angiography) in nearly every case, and have never seen a negative outcome from intercurrent embolization once heparin is instituted (112). Likewise, there is a small subset of patients with postoperative neurologic events (most often TIA) following CEA who are found to have a fresh thrombus adherent to the suture line (see Fig. 2-19), partially occluding the artery, and which is presumably the source of embolic phenomena. If there is no other angiographic evidence of technical inadequacy, I manage these patients conservatively as well, with full anticoagulation and six weeks follow-up arteriography (or, in the current era, MRA). In every case, the thrombus has resolved and there have been no negative neurologic outcomes in my series with this plan of management. Despite the surgeon's natural inclination to fix a problem with bold action, I have found that a measured conservative approach yields good results in cases of fresh or propagating thrombus and in my experience outweighs undertaking a high-risk surgical procedure.

Contralateral Carotid Occlusion

Early reports of surgery in the face of contralateral carotid occlusion were dismal (114), but with advances in surgical and anesthetic techniques, most surgeons currently have little or no hesitation to approach symptomatic carotid lesions with contralateral occlusion. Surgeons who employ selective shunting based on intraoperative monitoring do report a higher incidence of shunt-dependent cases in this group (115,116), and several studies have reported higher rates of postoperative neurologic deficits in this subgroup when shunts were not used (117,118). Several series dealing exclusively with this problem have been published, and all reported satisfactory results. Interestingly, three groups employed universal shunting in dealing with contralateral carotid occlusion (119–121), while the fourth reported excellent results in patients who were never shunted (122). It has been my policy to approach these cases with EEG monitoring and selective shunting, much as routine carotid procedures are performed, although unquestionably the need for intraluminal shunting has been greater in this subgroup. In my series where the shunt rate is ~15%, 25% of patients with contralateral occlusion have required shunts based on full-channel EEG criteria (123).

Notwithstanding my personal opinions on the safety of carotid surgery in patients with contralateral occlusion, we must note that NASCET data identified contralateral occlusion as an independent risk factor for poor outcome in reconstruction of symptomatic carotid disease (124). These data have been extensively cited in support of carotid stenting, as opposed to open surgery, for these purported "high-risk" patients.

There is new and compelling evidence to suggest that contralateral CEA is beneficial to both hemispheres in patients with symptomatic ICA occlusion. Rutgers and co-workers (125) showed that transcranial Doppler (TCD) flow increased bilaterally, basilar artery antegrade and ophthalmic artery reverse flow decreased, brain lactate levels decreased, and CO_2 reactivity increased following contralateral CEA when an occluded carotid was identified.

Tandem Lesions of the Carotid Siphon

The presence of carotid siphon disease has been proposed as a contraindication to CEA because of both the inability to pinpoint the symptomatic source and the reputed increased possibilities of postoperative occlusion from decreased carotid flow velocity. At least two surgical series have refuted these contentions (126,127). In both of these studies, no significant association between postoperative complications or recurrent symptoms could be demonstrated in patients undergoing CEA in the face of known "inaccessible" siphon disease. Several other interesting reports on this problem have been published. Day et al. (128) documented two cases of siphon disease resolution following ipsilateral CEA (128). Little et al. (129) described a similar entity of angiographic "pseudotandem stenosis," which likewise resolved in two cases following endarterectomy. The presence of a tandem lesion does not appear to contraindicate successful CEA if the indications and surgical risks are otherwise justified.

Intracranial atherosclerotic disease (IAD) was studied as an offshoot of NASCET. IAD was found to be an independent risk factor for stroke in medically treated NASCET patients and CEA reduces this risk (130).

Concurrent Carotid Disease and Intracranial Aneurysm

Several studies have focused on the repair sequencing of symptomatic carotid disease and silent intracranial aneurysm discovered on carotid angiography. Although one report documents rupture of an intracranial aneurysm six months following carotid reconstruction for tight stenosis (131), most other authors recommend repair of the symptomatic lesion first, which in most cases will be symptomatic carotid artery stenosis (132,133). These authors conclude that CEA is unlikely to precipitate rupture of intracranial aneurysm during the perioperative period.

A clever and elegant solution to the carotid/aneurysm dilemma, using a combined approach to both lesions at one operation, has been described by Hodge (134). This approach solves the waiting problem and merits consideration by surgeons with the ability to perform both techniques.

Recurrent Carotid Stenosis

A small but finite incidence of recurrent carotid stenosis occurs following primary CEA. Most authors quote a symptomatic recurrence rate of approximately 4% to 5%, and in one study of noninvasive follow-up after carotid surgery, a 4.8% recurrence rate of symptomatic carotid restenosis was documented with an additional 6.6% silent restenosis rate (135). Piepgras et al. (136) have quoted somewhat lower figures with their use of patchgraft repair (1% symptomatic, 4–5% total at two year follow-up).

Aside from technical inadequacies, it is difficult to identify risk factors associated with recurrent carotid stenosis, although continuation of smoking habits following endarterectomy proved to be a significant risk factor in one study whereas hypertension, diabetes mellitus, family history, lipid studies, aspirin use, and coronary disease were not found to be significant risk factors by this group (137,138).

Reoperation for carotid stenosis is a technically more difficult procedure than primary operation. Most surgeons feel that the stroke risk in redo CEA is associated with significantly higher risks than primary endarterectomy [4.8% vs. 0.8% in one recent series (139), 3.4% in another (140)], and the risk of cranial nerve injury is clearly increased as well. Piepgras et al. (136) carefully documented a reoperation CEA complication rate of 10.5%—four times their customary figure. At my institution, the possibility of reoperation for carotid stenosis is entertained for patients who present with angiographically proven disease and classical neurologic symptoms referable to the appropriate artery. In addition, since the ACAS data became available, we have routinely followed patients with noninvasive studies and recommended reoperation for high-grade recurrent stenosis when it is identified. Recurrent stenosis, however, was significantly reduced in my practice following the adoption of primary universal Hemashield patch angioplasty. We do see cases from other surgeons in which primary repair has failed, and we evaluate these patients in light of the ACAS data, taking special care to educate them of the higher risks associated with reoperative surgery when they make their surgical decision. The Mayo group likewise feels that changing bruits or rapidly progressive silent stenosis justifies surgical intervention (136).

Data from the SAPPHIRE trial now suggest that stenting should be considered as an equivalent therapy for "high-risk" carotid patients such as those with recurrent disease. It remains to be seen what paradigm will ultimately emerge regarding the endarterectomy/stenting balance for high-risk cases (141).

Concurrent Coronary/Carotid Disease

It is well established that patients with extracranial carotid artery disease have a higher than normal incidence of coronary disease as well as other peripheral vascular problems. Indeed, the risk of perioperative MI exceeds the risk of perioperative stroke in many clinical series of CEA. Several major questions arise when planning treatment for concurrent coronary/carotid disease. First—what is the risk of coronary revascularization in a patient with a high-grade asymptomatic stenosis or bruit; second—in patients with symptomatic carotid disease, what is the appropriate workup of the coronary circulation; and third—if both symptomatic carotid artery and coronary artery disease are identified, what is the appropriate surgical management of this patient: staged carotid followed by coronary revascularization, combined procedure, or "reverse-staged" coronary revascularization followed by delayed CEA.

The first of these questions regarding asymptomatic bruit in symptomatic coronary patients has been dealt with earlier in this chapter. We accept the ACAS evidence that suggests that carotid reconstruction is an appropriate choice for patients with 60% or greater stenosis. It is less clear whether carotid surgery is needed first for the asymptomatic bruit in patients about to undergo surgical procedures of a different type. In such cases, a reverse-staged strategy is appropriate. We reemphasize that symptomatic carotid disease is the harbinger of stroke in patients who are candidates for other surgery, and in cases of this type we recommend staged surgery with the carotid first.

The second question regarding appropriate workup of coronary disease in symptomatic carotid artery patients is a more difficult one. In this situation, workup is customarily guided by the patient's history and symptomatology. I obtain cardiology consultation for any patient with a history of angina, known heart disease, or abnormal resting electrocardiogram (ECG). The workup proceeds with a thallium stress test with exercise or dipyridamole, and if there is any evidence of myocardial ischemia, coronary angiography is performed (142,143).

When the results of cardiac evaluation indicate the need for coronary revascularization, the question becomes one of timing of the surgical procedures. I prefer to do staged procedures whenever possible. With careful hemodynamic monitoring and good anesthetic technique, I am routinely able to perform safe unilateral CEAs prior to coronary revascularization. The risks of combined procedures are high; Medicare population studies have documented a combined 17.7% stroke/death rate for combined CEA/CABG surgery, even though the majority of patients had asymptomatic carotid disease (144). An occasional patient with severe unstable angina may require a combined procedure, but clearly this entails a significantly higher surgical risk and I, like others with extensive experience, attempt staged procedures whenever possible (142,145). Most series dealing with "reverse stage" coronary carotid procedures (i.e., the coronary artery revascularization first with delayed CEA) discuss these in the context of asymptomatic carotid disease (146). In the first edition of this book I stressed my practice of not offering prophylactic revascularization to asymptomatic patients with or without concurrent coronary disease (9). Clearly, the ACAS/ACST results have changed our approach, and we now consider reverse-staged procedures an appropriate and effective strategy for risk reduction in patients who meet the ACAS criteria for prophylactic CEA (147).

TECHNICAL CONSIDERATIONS

Anesthesia Choice

The choice of anesthetic type for carotid reconstruction, whether local, regional, or general, is highly individualized by surgeon. It is also important to remember that monitoring, shunt philosophy, and anesthetic choice are intimately intertwined, and that the choice of local or regional anesthetic technique, at least in previous decades, implied the surgeon's belief that direct observation was an effective and probably the most accurate monitoring strategy to document cross-clamp ischemia and the consequent need for placement of an intraluminal shunt. In early reported series, however, failure to tolerate cross-clamping under regional anesthesia (RA) caused the procedure to be aborted (in 10% of cases), with a reoperation under general anesthesia (GA) and universal shunting 24 to 48 hours later (148). The current standard technique for local anesthesia (LA)/RA has evolved significantly, and this delay practice is no longer reported.

Local/Regional Anesthesia

It is difficult to ascertain with certainty the prevalence of LA/RA in carotid reconstruction. Despite a growing and renewed interest in the local/regional techniques, I think we can safely assume that GA remains the most common practice for carotid reconstruction across all specialties. In the NASCET randomized trial of symptomatic carotid disease (including both vascular and neurosurgeons), the majority (>95%) of patients underwent GA (149), and surprisingly only 55% were neurologically monitored. The later work of Cheng et al. (150) presents a survey of the members of the Society of Neuroanesthesia and Critical Care (SNACC). Of those who responded (50.7% of the surveyed group), 84.7% administered GA for CEA, while 16.7% used regional block anesthesia, and 2.8% reported either LA or a regional/general combination in their practices. These decisions, of course, were primarily made by the surgeon, but the data still should reflect accurately current neurosurgical practice since an anesthesia team will be present for all cases. Although the data are probably valid for neurosurgical CEA, it is unclear whether it can be extrapolated to the larger vascular/cardiothoracic population of surgeons, and whether the prevalence of LA/RA (which I suspect would be higher still) differs in those groups.

A discussion of local or regional carotid anesthesia is mostly academic for this author since I almost never use it in my practice (9,123,147,151–168). This is primarily because like many surgeons I am hesitant to deviate from a standardized operative plan (the use of essentially universal GA with full-channel EEG monitoring in my case) which has yielded good results. I have, on several occasions, performed successful CEAs under LA when the patients had pulmonary problems so severe that postoperative ventilator dependence was a risk.

Popular opinion on the use of LA changes in different surgical generations. External forces mandating decreased cost and length of stay by whatever means necessary may drive the surgical choice. Some have suggested that carotid surgery be performed essentially as an outpatient procedure (169) although I have reservations to this approach, particularly in patients with associated risk factors. I think we must say in fairness that the data reported by Harbaugh and Harbaugh (170) and Allen et al. (171) would indicate that significantly decreased morbidity, increased patient satisfaction, and complication rates equal to or better than the best general anesthetic series can now be demonstrated by surgeons committed to the local/regional anesthetic technique. Since the first edition of this book was published, compelling evidence has demonstrated that locoregional anesthesia is associated with significantly less perioperative hemodynamic instability than GA (172), and in a second, randomized trial, that LA patients with known ischemic heart disease had half the rate of perioperative myocardial ischemia as GA patients (173).

General anesthetics versus regional anesthetics have been directly compared in several recent series from single institutions (171,174–177). Forssell et al. (175) reported a randomized series of 101 patients in which 56 received LA and 55 received GA. There was no significant difference in stroke rate, but the rate of intraluminal shunt use (based on stump pressure for GA and neurologic observation for LA) was five-times higher in GA patients. LA patients, on the other hand, experienced significantly higher systemic blood pressure during cross-clamping (210 mmHg vs. 173 mmHg mean systolic) (175), Corson et al. reported 252 GA endarterectomies and 157 RA cases at Albany Medical Center (174). Monitoring in GA cases consisted of stump pressure and visual assessment of backbleeding; many patients under GA were shunted empirically. The stroke rate was significantly higher in the GA cases, and there was a higher incidence of labile blood pressure and the need for vasoactive drugs in the GA group. Five patients under RA required conversion to a general anesthetic. Allen et al. (171) made a strong case for the use of the regional technique. Their study compared 361 general anesthetic cases and 318 regional cases on the vascular surgical service at Washington University. There was no difference in stroke rate between anesthetic groups or between asymptomatic and symptomatic patients. Significantly more (42.1% vs. 19.2%) patients were shunted in the GA group than in the RA group. (Monitoring consisted of EEG plus stump pressure in GA cases and neurologic status observation in RA cases; patients with contralateral occlusion or recent stroke were shunted empirically in many cases.) RA patients had significantly shorter operative times, fewer perioperative cardiopulmonary complications, and shorter hospital stays. Shah et al. (178) revised and updated the earlier Albany series. In their study, RA reduced mean ICU stay from 1.4 to 0.7 days and hospital stay from 5 to 3 days. Palmer's community hospital study by a single surgeon using the two techniques disputes the length of stay and complications data, being unable to show a statistical difference (179).

It appears now that experienced surgeons who choose RA can apply it to all carotid patients they come across. This was not the case in earlier reports. There is good evidence from Harbaugh's series that the RA technique can be applied universally, eliminating the need, at least in his cases, for emergency intubation and/or procedure termination that complicated older reported series (170,180). Most current reports document little or no conversion to GA in patients operated with local/regional technique (181). It would appear that those rare cases where emergency induction of GA is required are primarily cases where airway control is inadequate following a severe neurologic change (unconsciousness) at cross-clamping, or for seizure occurring at cross-clamping (178). In Shah's report, 1.1% of patients required GA conversion, half for inadequate analgesia, and half for the aforementioned neurologic problems (178).

The implication of LA/RA is that the patient can be continually examined by either the anesthetist or surgeon or be required to perform some motor task (such as squeezing a child's toy with the contralateral hand) (182) to confirm adequate ipsilateral perfusion during cross-clamping. Groups with large experience in the technique report that the risk of patient disorientation from ischemia with subsequent movement and contamination of the operative field can be minimized by careful monitoring and sedation by the anesthetist (182–186). Proponents of LA stress the advantages of patient response to questioning as a superior monitoring technique in assessing the need for shunt placement, primarily because of dissatisfaction with the use of stump pressure measurements (186) or EEG monitoring (185) in the anesthetized patient. Other advocates of LA, including some who shunt routinely (184), report a 2% to 5% incidence of undetected shunt malfunction during endarterectomy (either from cephalad migration of the shunt with distal abutment against the ICA wall or from intraluminal thrombosis), and feel that direct observation of the awake patient is the most reliable indicator of shunt function (184,187). Perhaps, the most interesting data from the LA series are that of Steed et al. (183) who analyzed the causes of stroke during CEA in a series of 345 LA procedures. They found that intraoperative neurologic deficit was most often associated with dissection around the carotid (for exposure) or clamp reopening, and only rarely with carotid cross-clamping. Their data support the theory (also championed by those who never shunt) that most neurologic deficits are embolic rather than ischemic in nature.

We have recently analyzed our own institutional data, comparing the incidence of EEG changes and the need for shunting between two surgeons; a vascular surgeon who uses only LA/RA with EEG, and myself, using GA with EEG (176,177). In this series, the incidence of EEG changes and shunt placement was less with LA. There was no difference, however, in stroke rate, complications outcome, or length of stay.

The potential drawbacks of LA/RA for carotid reconstruction have been enumerated by Michenfelder (188). These include patient discomfort, the perceived need for hasty surgery and/or shunt placement, loss of patient cooperation if cross-clamp ischemia produces confusion, panic, or seizures, the possibility of a delayed deficit occurring at some time beyond the initial test period, the inability to administer cerebral protective (anesthetic) agents, and the inability to optimize blood gases and blood pressure to augment cerebral perfusion. It is difficult to document or discern from published reports the number of patients who are unable to tolerate the local/regional technique, but surgeons with great experience universally point out that extensive preoperative counseling and a skilled experienced anesthetist are the keys to preventing panic or lack of cooperation.

Either sequential infiltration of the cervical layers with 1% lidocaine or regional block anesthesia may be used for awake CEA. Hafner and Evans (189), reporting a series of 1200 CEAs, preferred local infiltration, with the feeling that regional block was not always successful in eliminating pain during cross-clamping. Other authors are satisfied with percutaneous cervical block anesthesia, although complications such as extension of anesthetic effect to the brachial plexus with transient monoparesis and generalized seizure (presumably from intra-arterial injection) have been documented (180,181). Mild sedation with midazolam hydrochloride is often added (189), and the need for block augmentation with local anesthetic infiltration is often mentioned (190). A complete description of the technique and its advantages can be found in Harbaugh's recent article (180).

Seizures at the time of cross-clamping, although rare, have been reported, leading to abandonment of the procedure (190) or as mentioned above conversion to a general anesthetic (178).

General Anesthesia

GA remains the technique of choice for carotid artery surgery in many centers for a number of reasons. Certainly, many surgeons prefer the more controlled surgical environment afforded by GA. It is my personal feeling that GA facilitates resident education, a fact that cannot be discounted. A light general anesthetic, mostly narcotic/N20 with a low concentration of inhalational agent, is commonly used. All commonly selected inhalational anesthetic agents, and intravenous barbiturates, significantly reduce $CMRO_2$ (191), providing a theoretical advantage in brain protection during ischemia. In addition, GA provides for accurate manipulation of respiratory parameters and arterial pCO_2, and facilitates rapid intraoperative control of blood pressure changes.

Manipulation of arterial pCO_2 to optimize cerebral protection has been the subject of great study and some debate. Intraoperative hypercapnia was initially felt to provide cerebral protection through vasodilation and increased global regional cerebral blood flow (rCBF) (192). Later investigations, however, showed that hypercapnia has no effect on either ipsilateral stump pressure (193) or rCBF (measured by gaseous washout) (194), and that indeed it may be deleterious (195). Hypocapnia, through the "inverse steal" effect (196–198), may be more effective in enhancing rCBF in ischemic areas (193, 195,196). One clinical study, however, in which patients were randomized into hypercapneic or hypocapneic techniques, could show no statistically significant difference in neurologic outcome between the two groups, although the hypocarbic group did have fewer neurologic complications (199). In view of these findings, patients undergoing carotid artery surgery are currently managed at normocapneic levels, or with only mild hyperventilation, avoiding extremes of arterial pCO_2 (191,200).

Data concerning induced-intraoperative hypertension is much more consistent. Significant increases in both local rCBF (194) and in stump pressure (191) have been documented with pharmacologically induced hypertension in patients undergoing carotid cross-clamping. Many surgeons, who shunt based on intraoperative monitoring, first attempt to reverse ischemic changes with a controlled elevation of arterial pressure. Cheng's data show that a majority of SNACC members use intraoperative hypertension (61.1%) routinely in carotid surgical anesthesia (150). Current anesthetic management in carotid surgery aims at maintenance of normotensive levels with tolerance of systolic pressure up to 20% higher before antihypertensive measures are instituted (19l). Certainly, it is also clear that intraoperative hypotension is to be avoided.

Monitoring Techniques During Carotid Cross-Clamping

The decision to perform endarterectomy, in my mind, implies that the surgeon will become familiar with and learn to rely on one specific monitoring technique to determine the need for shunt placement. (Basically, this is true for LA/RA as well, with the exception that the choice of monitoring style may not be quite as varied.) This opinion is not universally held. Some surgeons will shunt routinely, whether monitoring is used or not, and some will never shunt under the same conditions. There is, in my mind, no standard of care referable to the need for monitoring or the placement of a shunt. Nonetheless, in the ongoing attempt to reduce morbidity and mortality in carotid artery surgery under GA, a variety of intraoperative monitoring techniques have been developed to assess the need for increased cerebral protection, whether by induced hypertension or by intraluminal shunting. These techniques fall into two broad categories: (*i*) tests of vascular integrity, such as direct observation of backbleeding, stump-pressure measurements, xenon rCBF studies, TCD, intraoperative OPG, Doppler/duplex scanning, angiography, and near-infrared spectroscopy (NIRS), and (*ii*) tests of cerebral function, such as EEG, EEG derivatives, and/or SSEP monitoring. Monitoring techniques common to both LA/RA and GA include the cruder tests of vascular integrity (visual assessment, stump pressure) and the EEG/SSEP tests of neurologic function, as well as TCD. Direct assessment of patient response is of course only available under local/regional technique. Cheng's data indicate that 90% of SNACC responders used intraoperative neuromonitoring, with EEG being the most common method (67.5%) (150).

Monitoring Techniques Under GA

Vascular Evaluations

Visual Assessment of Backbleeding. Surgeons who may not have access to more sophisticated techniques of monitoring, and who choose to practice selective shunting, may rely on visual assessment of retrograde bleeding from the isolated ICA based on their experience. Although I make a quick assessment of backbleeding, my own practice is to assess the need for shunting based on EEG data.

Stump Pressure. Measurement of residual "stump" pressure in the isolated distal CCA or ICA following clamping of the proximal CCA and ECA was proposed as a simple and reliable indicator of the need for intraluminal shunting. The technique as described by Moore measured mean internal carotid back pressure, and most authors have subsequently adhered to this standard. In Moore's initial studies, mean stump values of greater than 25 mmHg were felt to represent the safe level for carotid back pressure (99,201), and they continue to advocate this method (202). Hays et al. and others later reported similar good results with this monitoring technique, but revised the safe level of mean arterial back pressure to 50 mmHg (203) or even as high as 70 mmHg (204). Others have emphasized that isolated stump-pressure measurements are not adequate, and recommend interpretation of such values in relation to the patient's resting blood pressure (205) or when jugular venous pressure was concurrently measured and the calculated cerebral perfusion pressure (CPP) was greater than 18 mmHg (206). Stump-pressure monitoring has come under criticism when evaluated simultaneously with other monitoring techniques. In two series of LA procedures, 6% to 9% of patients lost consciousness and required shunting despite stump pressures greater than 50 mmHg (207,208). In several general anesthetic series, stump pressures did not correlate well with either ischemic changes on EEG or with intraoperative rCBF measurements (209–213), and in one case, the incidence of ischemic changes on EEG despite stump pressures greater than 50 mmHg was 22% (209). At present, stump-pressure measurements, if taken, are usually augmented by evaluation of physiologic function in intraoperative evaluation of the need for shunting.

Intraoperative rCBF. Several centers have performed intraoperative rCBF analyses with intracarotid injection of ^{133}Xe; in some this remains a routine technique of assessment during carotid artery surgery (214–216). These studies have provided valuable information concerning both the lower limits of tolerable rCBF and concerning the correlation of rCBF values with EEG monitoring and stump-pressure data. Boysen originally felt that rCBF values of 30 cc/100 g/min represented the critical threshold for irreversible intraoperative ischemia (210). Later series, however, including Sundt's extensive experience, have revised this figure downward to 18–20 cc/100 g/min (213, 215–217). In most of these series, a good correlation has existed between failure of ipsilateral rCBF and slowing or flattening of the EEG, but several authors have stressed the lack of such correlation between rCBF and ipsilateral stump pressures (213,210). It is clear that most surgeons using rCBF determinations opt for intraluminal shunting at values below 18–20 cc/100 g/min. A single study, however, of patients in whom shunts were never used reports uneventful neurologic outcomes in some patients with intraoperative rCBF as low as 9 cc/100 g/min (218). These investigators are credible surgeons and their data must be taken seriously. Intraoperative rCBF studies have certainly provided valuable insights into cerebrovascular physiology, and in certain specialized centers continue to serve as a routine monitoring technique. Their value to the majority of carotid surgeons is limited by lack of availability of equipment and personnel trained in this methodology.

Transcranial Doppler. Continuous online recording of systolic and mean TCD velocities in the ipsilateral middle cerebral artery (MCA) during CEA is gaining increasing favor in the neurovascular surgical community. The advantages of TCD for carotid monitoring are several. These include the ability to predict the need for shunting by virtue of measuring a decrement in MCA velocities (MCAV), the ability to assess function of the shunt both after insertion (with an increase in MCAV) and during arterial repair (where presumably a shunt malfunction would manifest as a profound decrease in MCAV), and finally the ability to detect particulate embolization through audible TCD monitoring either during the procedure or in the postoperative period. We will examine each of these monitoring considerations in turn.

TCD may have the ability to predict preoperatively the need for shunting. Benichou et al. divided 91 patients into two groups. Group A patients had TCD identification of a functional anterior communicating and either one or two posterior communicating arteries preoperatively whereas Group B patients had no such communicating arteries identified. Group B patients had a significantly higher incidence of stump pressures <50 mmHg at surgery and clinical need for shunting. They found that the clinical need for shunting based on these preoperative criteria was correct in 95.6% of cases (219). Schneider et al. had likewise reported a similar statistically significant ability to predict decreased MCAV and shunt need in a somewhat smaller series of 23 patients (220). Sufficient experience with TCD now exists to allow the technique to be compared to other methods of intraoperative CEA monitoring. A number of papers have compared TCD monitoring with intraoperative stump-pressure measurements, customarily using a stump pressure of less than 50 mmHg as an indication for shunting (220–225). A good correlation with stump pressure and TCD monitoring has been reported although as one would suspect, TCD appears to be somewhat more sensitive and to be a more direct reflection of the status of intracranial circulation. Halsey studied TCD and rCBF in eight patients but found considerable variability in the relationship between the two (226). Thiel et al. studied TCD measurements and correlated these with intraoperative SSEP recordings. They used MCAV reduction of greater than 60% as their criterion for significant change in 78 patients. This degree of TCD decrease occurred 11 times, however, in only six of these patients did relevant SSEP changes occur simultaneously and one patient with critical SSEP changes did not have a significant MCAV reduction. The four patients, however, who did have transient neurological deficits postoperatively, had both critical MCA reduction and critical SSEP findings (227).

The correlation of intraoperative EEG with TCD has likewise been evaluated. Schneider et al. (220) showed that EEG changes occurred during cross-clamping in their patients with an MCAV of 14.7 compared with an MCAV of 24.1 in patients with normal intraoperative EEG tracing (220). Jorgensen (222) showed that a V_{mean}clamp: V_{mean} pre-clamp ratio below 0.4 was 97% effective in detecting essentially all patients with EEG flattening (222).

What is the value of TCD in predicting intraoperative cross-clamp ischemia and the need for shunting during carotid surgery? In the recent retrospective study by Halsey (228), 11 centers contributed 1495 CEAs monitored with TCD. The cases were divided into severe, mild, and no ischemia groups and both shunt use and perioperative stroke rates were assessed in these groups. Ischemia was defined as being severe if mean velocity in the first minute was 0% to 15% of pre-clamp value, mild if 16% to 40%, and absent if greater than 40%. Severe ischemia occurred in 7.2% of cases but cleared spontaneously in half. Persistent severe ischemia without shunt was associated with a high rate of severe stroke; this appeared to be prevented by shunt placement. As has been shown by Prioleau et al. (229), the stroke rate was actually higher with shunting in cases without severe ischemia (empirical shunting). A recent report by Jansen et al. likewise documented 130 consecutive operations in which severe ischemia (defined as a reduction of ≥70% MCAV) occurred in 16 patients. Concurrent severe EEG changes occurred in nine and were corrected by shunt use in eight and profound hypothermia in one (in a combined coronary/carotid procedure). These authors were encouraged by the value of TCD in predicting neurological outcome and the need for shunt placement (230).

Aside from the value of MCAV in predicting cross-clamp ischemia, acoustic feedback from the TCD is useful to assess continuing passage of intracranial emboli. TCD monitoring for circulating solid cerebral emboli with automated detectors has potential application in identifying patients with active but clinically silent extracranial embolic sources (cardiac, aortic, or carotid) who may then be treated prophylactically with warfarin or surgery, depending on the source (231). Transhemispheric passage of embolic material has been shown by TCD in patients with an active carotid plaque and contralateral carotid occlusion; the signals disappeared following CEA (232). Detection of intracranial embolization during various points of the carotid procedure has been discussed primarily by Spencer et al. who differentiate between air-bubble emboli and formed-element emboli, and likewise make a distinction between transient effects and ongoing emboli during long-term recording. Thirty-eight percent of their patients demonstrated air-bubble emboli at release of CCA cross-clamps. This was felt to be a relatively benign finding. Formed-element emboli were acoustically identical to air-bubble emboli but were defined as emboli that occurred during periods where no air-bubble emboli would be expected, i.e., not during release of cross-clamps or other similar operative times. Formed-element emboli were identified in 25% of patients and were associated with strokes and cerebral infarction when they persisted for several hours postoperatively, indicating presumably an arterial source for consistent platelet fibrin thrombi (233). Jansen et al. have also shown a significant relation between the number of embolic signals by TCD during surgical dissection of the carotid artery and the occurrence of intraoperative infarcts (234).

Finally, TCD has proven utility in preventing technical errors at surgery including malfunction of an indwelling shunt. A decrement in MCAV during the shunted portion of the endarterectomy with subsequent revision of shunt and return of velocity has been documented (235). Likewise, a case of perioperative restenosis due to intimal flap detected by MCAV decrease has been also reported (236). Powers and Smith (237) have also reported the utility of postoperative TCD recordings in documenting the course of a patient with severe carotid stenosis and thus a dysautoregulated hemisphere who developed hyperperfusion syndrome in the postoperative period (237).

Audible TCD signal can be used as an educational tool. Ackerstaff et al. documented higher audible embolic signals during various stages of CEA, and recommend that surgeons modify and refine their dissection and shunting techniques by using continuous audible feedback to reduce embolic events (238). Spencer documented significant reduction in operative stroke rates (7% decreasing to 2%) in a series of 500 patients where continuous TCD was used as an educational feedback tool (239).

In conclusion, increasing experience with TCD shows it to be an effective method of intraoperative monitoring, which has the potential to address several questions. These include cross-clamp ischemia and the need for shunting, evaluation of shunt function, and elimination of technical errors that yield particulate embolization during the surgical procedure. It would appear that the ability of TCD to evaluate perfusion pressure intracranially rather than at the carotid stump is a more accurate measure of the need for shunting.

Perioperative Retinal Arterial Pressure. Gee et al. studied retinal pressures intraoperatively to evaluate the efficacy of shunt placement. They showed clearly that an indwelling shunt appreciably elevated the ipsilateral ophthalmic systolic pressure over that noted during carotid clamping (240). Pearce et al. (241,242) have described a technique of supra orbital photoplethysomography that is said to provide immediate feedback concerning intraoperative shunt malfunction. In their small series (15 procedures), 20% of indwelling shunts were repositioned because of decreased intraoperative supra orbital artery flow. To my knowledge, however, neither of these plethysomographic methods is currently in common use.

Intraoperative Angiography. A single intraoperative common carotid angiogram can be obtained following arterial closure and has been long championed by several groups (243–247). The methodology has been well described and involves puncture of the proximal CCA with hand injection of 10 mL of contrast while a single portable image is obtained (243). Radiographic defects requiring revision of the arterial suture line are demonstrated in 2.5% and 8% (246,247) of procedures in these series, and the authors feel neurologic sequelae have been markedly reduced by the ability to immediately assess the surgical site. The educational value of routine intraoperative angiography is also useful for facilitating error recognition and promoting continuous refinement of surgical technique (246,248).

The primary disadvantage of intraoperative angiography is one of time and convenience. All authors emphasize that these factors are reduced with consistency of radiographic personnel and increased experience on the surgeon's part. One group also feels that the risk of subintimal injection and consequent thrombosis outweighs the benefits of the technique in routine cases, and recommends that the arteriogram be reserved only for use when some question exists about the status of the arterial repair (such as distal intimal tacking, obvious external stenosis, or difficult distal shunt placement) (249). This position has been challenged by Blaisdell (243), who routinely uses arteriography and has not encountered a subintimal injection problem. At present, intraoperative completion arteriography seems to enjoy favor among surgeons familiar with the technique, but is not the standard of care.

A potential application of intraoperative angiography has been suggested in cases where patients awaken with a new neurological deficit. The patient is returned to the operating room, the wound is opened, and a hand injection of contrast media is performed while taking a single cervical x-ray. Gross technical errors or thrombosis can be identified by this technique without the need for reopening the vessel or the delay of proceeding to the angiographic suite.

Intraoperative Doppler Scanning. Informal use of sterilized Doppler probes applied to all vessels in the arteriotomy tree is commonly employed as a qualitative measure of postarteriotomy patency. I have used this method to demonstrate audible patency following carotid reconstruction, and like others (250) have used the Doppler to auscultate flow through an indwelling shunt. Formal Doppler or duplex scanning intraoperatively is also used. One study of Doppler spectrum analysis in 45 carotids imaged both pre- and postendarterectomy was useful in detecting technical errors and in predicting the need for intraoperative arteriography (251). In two others, intraoperative Doppler analysis demonstrated ICA defects in 4.3% to 4.5% of arteries and ECA abnormalities in 8.7% to 9% (187,252).

Functional Evaluations

EEG Monitoring. Intraoperative assessment of the EEG has withstood the test of time as a popular, readily available, and reliable method for determining cross-clamp dependent ischemia and the need for indwelling shunt. While early investigators merely correlated EEG changes observed at surgery (in non-shunted patients) with postoperative neurological deficits (253), EEG monitoring rapidly gained favor and was shown by several groups to correlate well with the need for shunting in both awake (254) and anesthetized (217,250,255–257) patients. The number of patients who show EEG changes during carotid clamping has varied according to different series: being as low as 8.5% (257) or as high as 31% (253). In my own series, 15% of patients have EEG changes and shunt placement. This increases to 25% if contralateral carotid occlusion is present (9,163–166). The ability of angiographic findings to predict intraoperative EEG changes has been low (258,259), and even patients with contralateral carotid occlusion, although appearing to require shunts more often than routine cases, have shown EEG changes in only 17% and 42%, respectively, in two series (115,116).

The EEG changes associated with intraoperative ischemia have been well documented, and consist most often of generalized slowing and decreased amplitude in the ischemic hemisphere (217,253,256,260). Chiappa has proposed that attenuation of anesthetic-induced fast rhythms may be more significant than ipsilateral slowing of the EEG and recommends that the electroencephalograph sensitivity be sufficient to monitor this fast activity (261). Trojaborg and Boysen (217) also measured simultaneously the intraoperative EEG and ipsilateral rCBF. They showed that EEG slowing correlated with rCBF values of 16 to 22 mL/100 g/min (227), whereas flattening of the EEG occurred with values of 11 to 19 cc/100 g/min. Several groups have documented EEG changes developing with intraoperative hypotension and have stressed avoidance of this complication (255,257).

Despite the inclination of many surgeons to shunt patients who have so-called moderate EEG changes as defined by Blume et al. (262), it should be recognized that there are investigators who do not share this viewpoint. Blume et al. studied 176 consecutive patients undergoing CEA without shunt. Nineteen percent of their patients had moderate EEG changes and 22 had "major EEG changes." Despite their lack of shunt use, there were no postoperative strokes in either the EEG unchanged or EEG moderately changed groups. Nine percent of patients with major clamp-associated EEG changes did develop postoperative strokes in their study.

Computerized EEG processing techniques have been developed to quantitate the information the EEG contains and display it in a format readily accessible to the surgical and anesthetic teams, eliminating the necessary presence in the operating room of personnel trained in electroencephalographic interpretation. Such displays typically provide trend analysis and provide rapid evaluation of the EEG under intraoperative conditions. Most computerized EEG analysis techniques convert the EEG from the time domain to the frequency domain. In the conversion process, amplitude, measured in voltage, is changed to a derivative of voltage—power. Compressed spectral array (CSA) and density-modulated spectral array (DSA) are two ways of displaying this power spectrum analysis. Several parameters have been derived to simplify the description and interpretation of these complex displays of frequency and power data. The three most commonly used are the median power frequency (MPF), the frequency at the median of the power spectrum; the peak power frequency (PPF), the frequency comprising the largest single component of the power spectrum; and the spectral edge frequency (SF) the highest frequency in the power spectrum in which there is activity. These systems are attractive, appear to yield good results, and will certainly undergo continuing refinement (261,263–267).

SSEP Monitoring. Considerable interest has been generated in the use of median nerve generated SSEP as predictors of cerebral ischemia, reflected both as the need for intraoperative shunting or as a predictor of poor neurologic postoperative outcome. Several important questions exist regarding SSEP monitoring during CEA. These include the criteria to be used for SSEP prediction of neurologic events, questions regarding the false positive and false negative rate of the technique, and finally whether the technique is sufficient to supersede the more standard electrophysiologic technique of online EEG discussed previously.

SSEP criteria for cross-clamp cerebral ischemia include either prolongation of the central conduction time (latency) or reduction in amplitude of the SSEP. Most authors have used 50% amplitude reduction of the N20-P25 SSEP as their criterion for specifying significant cerebral ischemia (200,268–276). Others have used a bimodal technique whereby either a prolongation of central conduction time or a decreased SSEP amplitude represent event criteria (277). No matter which criteria are used to determine the need for shunting, however, it is clear that complete loss of amplitude, i.e., flat SSEP is associated with a profound postoperative neurological deficit in 100% of cases where responses do not return with or without shunting (268,269,278). The entire subject of SSEP monitoring during carotid surgery has been well reviewed by Markand (260).

The literature varies widely regarding the rates of false positive and false negative results with the use of the SSEP technique. Several authors report a false positive rate of zero when SSEP flattening is the criterion (i.e., as mentioned, all patients with irreversible SSEP loss had a neurologic deficit) (269–272,279), whereas at 50% amplitude decrease level, Lam et al. reported many false positives (275). False positives exist with many monitoring techniques, however, and are not unique to SSEP recording. The more serious question of whether or not false negatives exist is also debated. Although Amantini et al. (268,269) reported no false negatives (i.e., no cases in which neurological deficit ensued with normal SSEP tracings throughout), some false negative outcomes (admittedly rare) have been reported by others including De Vleeschauwer (270) in 3/177 cases, Horsch (272) in 4/586 cases, and Haupt (271) in 1/994 cases. Two recent articles elucidate best the current level of the debate regarding SSEP monitoring during CEA. The study of Tiberio et al. (276) included 264 surgical procedures with criteria for shunt insertion being central conduction time prolongation greater than 1 msec and/or N20-P25 amplitude decrease of at least 50%. Eighty-nine percent of cases had normal SSEP and 11% had abnormal SSEP. A shunt was used in 9% of cases and no patient had a permanent neurological deficit. These authors argue strongly that SSEP is a highly reliable predictor of the need for shunting and use it as their primary monitoring technique. In direct contradistinction to this is the recent article by Kearse et al. (274), who monitored simultaneously the EEG and SSEP in 53 CEAs. Rather than using neurological outcome as an endpoint, their SSEP criteria were measured against EEG as a "gold standard," and in their 23 patients with EEG evidence of ischemia following cross-clamping, 10 had prolongation of the central conduction time but only one had an amplitude decrease of 50% or greater. It was their strong conclusion that SSEP was not sufficiently sensitive to reliably identify compromised cerebral perfusion that was readily discernible by EEG in these cases (274).

We should finally mention one interesting case report by Gautier et al. in which online monitoring of SSEP showed a loss of amplitude during head positioning in preparation for CEA (280). In this case, SSEP disappeared eight minutes following head positioning consisting of neck extension and rotation of the head to the right. Return of the head to a neutral position resulted in a normalization of SSEP and the surgical procedure was then completed uneventfully.

NIRS Measurement. The latest monitoring technique introduced is continuous monitoring of cerebral hemoglobin oxygen saturation by NIRS techniques (281,282). This technique uses a simple probe applied to the forehead to measure oxyhemoglobin (oxy-Hb), deoxyhemoglobin (deoxy-Hb), and total hemoglobin continuously, with special attention paid to changes in their ratio during cross-clamping, clamp release, and with or without shunt insertion. Kirkpatrick et al. (281) reported good correlation between increased deoxy-Hb, decreased oxy-Hb, and a rapid fall in MCAV by simultaneous TCD measurement at the time of cross-clamping (281). Kuroda et al. (282) correlated NIRS with rCBF [by single photon emission computed tomography (SPECT)] and with SSEP measurements. They describe two classes of patients; in the first, initial decrease in oxy-Hb/increase in deoxy-Hb corrects rapidly and spontaneously in the first few minutes after cross-clamping, these patients do not show SSEP or rCBF changes. In the second group, the NIRS changes are more rapid and sustained following clamping, and are associated with profound decreases in rCBF and loss of N20 amplitude on SSEP; in this group the changes do not reverse until an indwelling shunt is placed (282). Clearly, the technique of NIRS measurement to determine the need for shunt placement holds promise, but further validation studies will need to be performed before it is widely available or accepted. Kirkpatrick has discussed NIRS and its potential weaknesses in great detail (281,283,284).

Intraoperative Shunting

The necessity for indwelling arterial shunt during CEA is one of the most widely debated and long-standing controversies in neurovascular surgery. Carotid surgeons generally group themselves into three; those who use shunts in every case, those who employ shunting when indicated by some form of intraoperative monitoring, and those who never shunt no matter what the clinical or monitoring situation. My personal preference is to use a custom shunt of my own design (285) (Loftus shunt, Integra Neuroscience, Plainsboro, NJ), which is secured in the ICA with a special encircling type clamp (Loftus shunt clamp, Scanlan Medical Instruments, St. Paul, MN). Aufiero et al. (286) have discussed the performance characteristics associated with different shunt choices in detail (286).

Monitoring is most critical for surgeons who practice selective (monitoring-dependent) shunt placement, as I do. For those who have chosen to shunt every case, or for those who never place a shunt, intraoperative monitoring, while interesting, will not customarily affect treatment decisions, and may not be used at all. Likewise, surgeons who prefer shunting may practice in settings where monitoring is not available, and may thus choose universal shunting to afford maximum theoretical protection against cross-clamp ischemia.

Proponents of universal shunting argue that their technique is benign, assures the maximum degree of cerebral protection in every case, and eliminates dependence on specialized intraoperative monitoring techniques (120,287–291). They emphasize the relaxed surgical environment afforded by shunt flow and feel that extra time can be taken to ensure meticulous attention to the intimal dissection and arteriotomy repair. Some also point out the value of the shunt tubing as a stent to aid arterial closure (287).

Those who argue against routine intraluminal shunting do so on several grounds. They feel strongly that shunt placement is not nearly so benign, and carries with it the risks of distal particulate embolization. In one series, the stroke incidence in shunted cases was actually far higher than in a nonshunted control series (229). Occult shunt malfunction, whether from thrombosis, distal clamping, or distal abutment against the internal carotid wall, has been mentioned by several authors and may be more common than generally realized (182,184,292), and with few exceptions (292) there are currently no effective direct means available to monitor shunt flow. The possibility of distal intimal damage from the shunt end leading to embolization or carotid dissection is also present (293). Because of these risks, numerous nonshunting series have been accumulated and published. Gross et al. (294) successfully substituted barbiturate-induced burst suppression for shunt placement in cases where EEG changes did not respond to hypertensive therapy, but this method has not been accepted widely (294). Spetzler has likewise reported excellent nonshunted results with a strategy of intraoperative barbiturates and microsurgical technique (295). Several large series have been presented where good surgical results are obtained without shunt placement under any circumstances (117,296–303). These authors do not deny the existence of postoperative stroke, but they feel strongly that neurologic deficits from carotid surgery are invariably embolic rather than hemodynamic in nature, and that intraoperative monitoring and/or shunt placement will not further reduce the already low morbidity in their series (298). Ferguson (301), who has been perhaps the foremost advocate of nonshunting, has indicated that he does feel shunting may be of value in a very small percentage of cases with "severe" EEG changes and stump pressures of 25 mmHg or less.

Nearly all authors, even those who shunt routinely, agree that shunts are probably not required in the majority of carotid procedures (304). The merits and wisdom of selective shunting based on intraoperative monitoring criteria, and the impressive results with this technique in a large series of patients, have been well documented by Sundt (214,216).

It should finally be noted that a number of authors who customarily advocate selective shunting have found intraoperative monitoring to be unreliable in patients having had recent reversible ischemic neurologic deficit (RIND) or stroke. These groups recommend empirical shunt placement in all such cases (98,99,305). On the contrary, Green et al. (306) reviewed their series of selective shunting, and felt that the benefit of EEG monitoring was in protecting the patient from the risky insertion of a shunt. They argued that there was no benefit from selective shunting (over nonshunting) unless the patient had sustained a recent stroke prior to surgery (306).

Is the Shunt Needed?

It should be clear that shunt use is an individual surgeon's choice. The need for intraoperative shunting, as discussed more extensively above and as described by published monitoring techniques, can be summarized as follows:

- Awake: deficit within 60 seconds
- Stump: carotid stump back pressure <50 mmHg
- CPP: stump-IJP <18 mmHg
- rCBF: 18–20 mL/100 g/min
- TCD: MCAV 0% to 15% preclamp
- EEG: unilateral attenuation 8–15 Hz fast or 2× increase 1 Hz delta
- SSEP: 50% amplitude decrease or 5% to 20% latency increase in central conduction time
- NIRS: rapid increase in deoxy-Hb, decrease in oxy-Hb, without return.

Insertion of the Shunt

The technique for insertion of an indwelling shunt varies among surgeons and is based on the type of shunt used. The basic principles I use to place a shunt can be summarized as follows:

- Total exposure above plaque
- Shunt in CCA first
- Evacuation of shunt
- Gentle ICA insertion
  - Backbleeding allowed
  - Shunt open to distend ICA lumen
- Doppler of shunt to auscultate flow
- Monitoring must return

These techniques are discussed and illustrated in detail in the second section (see Fig. 3-43 to 3-52).

Is the Shunt Working?

Similarly, the shunt, once placed, needs to carry blood and ensure cerebral perfusion. This can be ascertained in several ways, depending on the monitoring technique chosen by the surgeon, as follows:

- Functional evaluations—recovery of EEG, SSEP, or NIRS
- Vascular evaluations—return of MCAV by TCD, return of rCBF, Doppler auscultation of shunt.

MCAV and TCD criteria with specific shunt types have been elegantly addressed by Hayes et al. (307), who feel that performance is optimized by the Pruitt–Inahara design (307). Whether a complete return of MCAV to baseline during shunting is needed is less clear.

Arteriotomy Techniques

Some areas of controversy exist concerning technical performance of the carotid arterial repair. Objective data on these subjects is scarce owing to the difficulty of attributing success or failure in large series of patients to skill variance among surgeons. A few topics, however, are worthy of mention.

Patch Grafting

Most surgeons favor patch grafting the internal carotid repair in cases of recurrent stenosis, and many employ patch grafts selectively in a primary repair where the internal carotid lumen has been sufficiently narrowed to cause concern about postoperative stenosis and possible thrombosis. The routine use of patch grafts has been advocated by Little et al., who present data that show a statistically significant decrease in postoperative occlusion between grafted and nongrafted groups (308). Since the first edition of this book was published, several new studies provide further compelling evidence for the superiority of primary patch graft angioplasty versus simple primary closure. This evidence includes individual case series from experienced surgeons such as Archie, who reports a statistically significant decrease in restenosis/reoperation when patch grafting is used (309), multivariate analysis of multistate Medicare outcome data, in which patch grafting, intraoperative Heparin, and perioperative aspirin produced statistically better outcomes (310), and at least one randomized clinical trial, in which patch closure was less likely to cause ipsilateral stroke, TIAs, or recurrent carotid stenosis (311,312).

The choice of material, whether venous or synthetic, appears to be of little consequence. Yamamoto et al. felt strongly that synthetic materials were superior to sapenous vein because of the fear of aneurysm formation and central vein patch rupture (313). Several other studies have shown no effective difference between synthetic and vein patch in postoperative stroke rate; admittedly these studies did not address the question of central patch rupture (312,314,315). One recent randomized trial does appear to show an advantage in prevention of perioperative stroke, carotid thrombosis, and early restenosis when polytetraflouroethylene (PTFE) patches are used instead of collagen-impregnated Dacron (Hemashield); one offsetting disadvantage is the longer time to hemostasis needed for PTFE (316).

Although I previously reserved patch grafting for reoperative carotids, I have now adopted a policy of universal roof patch angioplasty with the Hemashield graft. Since adoption of this policy about eight years ago, and with routine postoperative interval duplex scanning, my incidence of significant (amenable to surgery) recurrent stenosis under observation has dropped to almost nothing.

Tacking Sutures

The use of tandem sutures to secure the distal intima in the internal carotid has been deemed unnecessary by some (289,299,317) yet has been cited by others as one of the major technical improvements in reducing carotid surgical morbidity (288). Although such sutures have the potential to narrow the internal carotid lumen, this risk seems low in comparison to the possibility of intimal dissection if a loose flap is left behind. Patterson (120) and Ferguson (299), among others, point out that tacking sutures become unnecessary if the ICA is carried far enough to visualize normal intima distal to the plaque. These arguments are reasonable; however, experienced carotid surgeons agree, even with excellent ICA exposure, that in some cases a clean distal endpoint cannot be achieved, and if there is any question of potential subintimal dissection, I place distal tacking sutures (in approximately 10% of cases), usually at the 4- and 8 O'clock positions.

Heparinization

Intravenous heparin is routinely administered at some point prior to arterial cross-clamping and repair. The dose, which may vary from 2500 to 10,000 units, is a matter of individual preference. One group has suggested a weight-based dosing schedule of 85 mg/kg with good results (318). Many surgeons (317) reverse the intraoperative anticoagulation with protamine at the conclusion of surgery, and Chandler has shown that reversal of this heparinization does not produce increased carotid thrombogenicity in dog carotids (319). Others, including myself, do not reverse the anticoagulation.

There is no evidence that this single dose of anticoagulant contributes to intraoperative or postoperative bleeding any more than the preoperative antiplatelet or anticoagulant agents most carotid patients receive, and there is compelling evidence that protamine use increases the stroke rate (320). Indeed, Gross et al. (294) validated a common practice when they reported a series of patients with threatened stroke in whom endarterectomy was performed under full systemic anticoagulation; no untoward problems with the arterial repair were encountered (294). I do not hesitate to operate with full heparinization throughout the procedure in patients with crescendo TIAs.

For several years, we have adopted a policy of checking intraoperative ACT during anesthesia induction in patients who are heparinized preoperatively. Almost invariably the anticoagulation is subtherapeutic and an additional tailored bolus dose is required at cross-clamping time.

SURGICAL TECHNIQUE OF CERVICAL CAROTID RECONSTRUCTION

Only surgeons with excellent perioperative morbidity and mortality results can offer carotid patients an outcome superior to the best available medical management. In this section, a technical scheme for CEA is presented that has yielded a combined morbidity and mortality of 2% (inclusive of patients in all risk grades including recent stroke) in my hands, and which allows me to confidently recommend carotid surgery to appropriate patients. I fully recognize that different techniques have proven successful for individual surgeons, and eschew a dogmatic approach to carotid surgery. It has proven valuable in my practice, however, to perform all carotid surgery with a uniform technical approach, thereby avoiding oversights or the necessity of hurried intraoperative decisions, and I present here an overview of the methods I have found most useful. Refer to part 3 for an illustrated, step-by-step description of the technique.

Indications

I have summarized earlier the data from the major randomized carotid indications trials. My policy regarding indications for surgery is to follow the recommendations of the large randomized cooperative trials and of the most recent AHA Guidelines (32). I propose surgery for all asymptomatic patients with linear stenosis of ≥60%, since this was the group that was shown to benefit from surgery in the ACAS trial (10). The benefit is not as great for women, and the benefit depends on the ability to perform surgery with a combined morbidity/mortality of less than 3%. Patients need to have an expected survival of five years following surgery to benefit from CEA if they are asymptomatic; for this reason patients with malignancies or other life-threatening conditions should not be offered surgery.

Patients with symptomatic carotid stenosis, whether evident as TIA or stroke, benefit from surgery if their arteriogram shows ≥50% linear stenosis as measured by the NASCET method (69,70) (see below). This benefit is greatest in men who are non-diabetic (diabetes clearly increases the surgical risk). According to several carotid trials (69,71,74), the benefit is realized immediately, so there should be no delay in operating on such patients. The benefit of surgery is also greatest in patients who have hemispheric symptoms instead of amaurosis fugax, and patients with plaque ulceration are at higher risk than those with smooth plaques (Fig. 1). We offer surgery to nearly all patients with symptoms and ⩾50% linear stenosis.

It is still unclear what treatment is best for ulcerated plaques (which intuitively would seem more dangerous) of less than 50% and for recurrent stenosis, whether symptomatic or asymptomatic. We sometimes offer surgery for deep ulcers of less than 50% stenosis, especially if they have hemispheric symptoms. We offer surgery for recurrent stenosis when symptoms are present, and also for patients who rapidly progress to high-grade stenosis while being followed with serial noninvasive studies. The risk of surgery is of course higher in cases of recurrent stenosis, and the patient must be informed of this. In the current era, an endovascular approach should also be considered for recurrent disease, although the results are unproven.

Preoperative Studies and Preparation

Patients with acute ischemic strokes or TIAs undergoing workup for their stroke etiology should have bilateral carotid duplex studies or MRA. Asymptomatic patients who on clinical evaluation are noted to have a carotid bruit or significant atherosclerotic disease should undergo similar testing. The population of patients with a documented lesion in either study should proceed to a tailored arteriogram (arch and both carotids, cervical and cranial), which at our institution still remains the gold standard for preoperative evaluation for CEA. The stenosis is defined from the NASCET criteria, where N is the linear diameter at the area of greatest narrowing, and D is the greatest diameter of the normal artery distal to the carotid bulb.

$$\text{Percent (\%) stenosis} = (1 - N/D) \times 100$$

Preoperative evaluation also involves aggressive workup of any patients with cardiac symptoms before CEA is performed.

Patients taking aspirin preoperatively are instructed to continue their therapy without interruption. Patients taking clopidrogel (Plavix®) or ticlopidine (Ticlid®) are switched to a daily aspirin one week before surgery (this strategy markedly reduces intraoperative oozing associated with these drugs). Patients on warfarin anticoagulation therapy for artificial heart valves, TIAs, and other indications (crescendo TIAs or critical stenosis) should be preoperatively admitted to the hospital and have their iatrogenic coagulopathy converted to IV heparin therapy. The heparin should be continued to the operating room and is stopped when the arterial closure is complete. As mentioned, some patients require postoperative heparin infusion for mechanical cardiac valves; these patients should be considered high-risk patients. We do not use protamine for reversal of anticoagulation.

Surgical Technique

In my opinion, there are several cardinal principles for carotid reconstruction

- Complete knowledge of the patient's vascular anatomy.
- Complete vascular control at all times.
- Anatomical knowledge to prevent harm to adjacent structures.
- Assurance of a widely patent repair free of technical errors.

It is our feeling that the meticulous anatomical dissection and identification of vital cervical structures needed to minimize postoperative complications can be achieved only with a bloodless field. Accordingly, we do not consider elapsed time to be a factor in the performance of carotid surgery. On our service, CEA requires from two to two-and-a-half hours of operating time and the average cross-clamp time is between 30 and 40 minutes. No untoward effects from the length of the procedure have been observed in any patients and we are convinced that the risk of cervical nerve injury or postoperative complications related to hurried closure of the suture line are significantly reduced by meticulous attention to detail.

The author has developed a complete set of custom carotid instruments (see Fig. 3-1) (Scanlan Instruments, St. Paul, MN), which we use in every case. The improvements in this set include two sizes of well-balanced vascular pickups, special dissecting scissors for coarse and fine work, and specialized cross-clamps, shunt clamps, and needle drivers. Microring-tip forceps are included as well to clean small fragments from the artery prior to repair. The beauty of a single set that includes everything needed for the operation cannot be overstated.

Two surgeons trained in the procedure are always present during carotid surgery. Both surgeons may stand on the operative side, the primary surgeon facing cephalad and the assistant facing the patient's feet (this is our preference), or the surgeons may stand on either side of the table. The operative nurse may stand either behind or across the table (in our setup) from the primary surgeon. The patient is positioned supine on the operating room table with the head extended and turned away from the side of operation. Several folded pillowcases are placed between the shoulder blades to facilitate extension of the neck and the degree of rotation of the head is determined by the relationship of the external and ICA on preoperative angiography. The carotid vessels are customarily superimposed in the antero-posterior plane, and moderate rotation of the head will swing the internal carotid laterally into a more surgically accessible position. In those patients where the internal carotid can be seen angiographically to be laterally placed, the head rotation need not be that great. On the other hand, occasional patients will demonstrate an internal carotid that is rotated medially under the external carotid, and in such cases no degree of head rotation will yield a satisfactory exposure. In these cases, the surgeon must be prepared to mobilize the external carotid more extensively and swing it medially to expose the underlying internal carotid (even tacking it up to medial soft tissues if necessary) (see Figs. 3-4 and 3-26).

The position of the carotid bifurcation has been likewise determined before surgery from the angiogram and the skin incision is planned accordingly. We always use a vertical type linear incision along the anterior portion of the sternomastoid muscle. This may go as low as the suprasternal notch and as high as the retro-aural region depending on the level of the bifurcation. The skin and subcutaneous tissues are divided sharply to the level of the platysma, which is always identified and divided sharply as well. Hemostasis often requires generous use of electrocautery. Self-retaining retractors are then placed and the underlying fat is dissected to identify the anterior edge of the sternocleidomastoid muscle. Retractors are left superficial at all times on the medial side to prevent retraction injury to the laryngeal nerves, but laterally may be more deeply placed. Dissection proceeds in the midportion of the wound down the sternomastoid muscle until the jugular vein is identified. Care must be taken under the sternomastoid muscle, however, to prevent injury to the spinal accessory nerve, which can be inadvertently transected or stretched.

We emphasize that the jugular vein is the key landmark in this exposure and complete dissection of the medial jugular border should always be carried out before proceeding to the deeper structures. [A fascinating retrojugular approach to the carotid has been described; I personally have not tried this technique (321).] In some corpulent individuals, the vein is not readily apparent and a layer of fat between it and the sternomastoid must be entered to locate the jugular itself. If this is not done, it is possible to fall into an incorrect plane lateral and deep to the jugular vein. As soon as the jugular is identified, dissection is shifted to come along the medial jugular border (antejugular approach) and the vein is held back with blunt retractors. The importance of the blunt retractor in preventing vascular injury at this point cannot be overemphasized. In this process, several small veins and one large common facial vein are customarily crossing the field and need to be doubly ligated and divided. The underlying carotid artery is soon identified once the jugular is retracted. Most often we come upon the CCA first and at the point of first visualization, the anesthesiologist is instructed to give 5000 units of intravenous heparin that is never reversed. Many surgeons routinely use intraoperative ACT to ensure that an adequate level of anticoagulation has been achieved with a goal of doubling the ACT. We have adopted this practice for patients who are brought to surgery on continuous heparin, and find that in such cases the ACT often confirms subtherapeutic heparinization, requiring a supplemental bolus dose. Poisik et al. (318) have also recently suggested a clever weight-based dosing system for heparin. Dissection of the carotid complex is then straightforward, and the CCA, ECA, and ICA are isolated with the gentlest possible dissection and encircled with "0" silk ties (or vessel loops if preferred) passed with a right-angle clamp. We do not routinely inject the carotid sinus, however, we notify the anesthesiologist when the bifurcation is being dissected, and if any changes in vital signs ensue (this is very rare), the sinus is injected with 2 to 3 cc of 1% plain xylocaine through a short 25 g needle. Although the carotid complex is completely exposed, the common and external carotids are not dissected free from their underlying beds in order to prevent postoperative kinking and coiling of these vessels. We dissect these arteries circumferentially only in those areas where silk ties or clamps are placed around them. Posterior dissection is more extensive in the region of ICA, where posterior tacking sutures may be placed later and tied.

The common carotid silk or an umbilical tape is passed through a wire loop that is then pulled through a rubber sleeve (Rummel tourniquet) thereby facilitating constriction of the vessel around an intraluminal shunt if this becomes necessary. The external and internal carotid ties or loops are merely secured with mosquito clamps. Particular attention is paid to the superior thyroid artery, which is dissected free and secured with a double loop "0" silk ligature (some prefer an aneurysm clip for this). A hanging mosquito clamp keeps tension on this occlusive Pott's tie. Occasionally, multiple branches of this artery are identified on the preoperative angiogram and these must be individually dealt with so that no troublesome backbleeding will ensue during the procedure through ignorance of these vessels. It is also essential that the external carotid silk tie (and subsequent cross-clamp) be placed proximal to any major external branches, lest unacceptable backbleeding occur during the arteriotomy and repair.

Proper placement of the retractors facilitates the control of the carotid system. The hanging mosquitoes and silk ties are draped over these retractor handles to keep the field uncluttered. We are especially fond of the blunt hinged modified Richards mastoid retractor, which is invaluable in exposing the ICA when a far distal exposure is necessary.

The dissection of the ICA must be complete and clearly beyond the distal extent of the plaque before cross-clamping is performed. A clear plane can be developed if the jugular vein is followed distally and dissection follows the plane between the lateral carotid wall and the medial jugular border. By following this plane, the hypoglossal nerve is readily identified as it swings down medial to the jugular and crosses toward the midline over the internal carotid. We have found it preferable to mobilize the nerve along its lateral wall adjacent to the jugular vein, after which it can be isolated with a vessel loop and gently retracted from the field, in this way we always know its position and will not inadvertently grasp the nerve with forceps, coagulate it, or transect it. With this technique, hypoglossal paresis is rare and seems to result instead in cases where the nerve is not visualized and is blindly retracted. Occasionally, adequate mobilization of the hypoglossal nerve requires ligation of a small arterial branch of the external carotid to the sternocleidomastoid muscle that loops over the nerve. We have never seen nor caused inadvertent (or advertent) transection of the hypoglossal nerve.

There are several other nerves that can be injured during carotid exposure and endarterectomy. The spinal accessory and hypoglossal nerves have already been discussed. The vagus nerve lies deep to the carotid in the carotid sheath and can be inadvertently cross-clamped if not identified. The marginal mandibular branch of the facial nerve can be stretched by medial retraction in the high exposure of the internal carotid, and the greater auricular nerve is at risk in a high incision, leaving the patient with a troublesome numb ear if it is transected. We have seen Horner's syndrome (always transient) from unrecognized injury to the peri-carotid sympathetic chain. Cutaneous sensory nerves will always be transected with the skin incision, and we advise patients that the anterior triangle of their neck will be numb for about six months following endarterectomy, after which sensation customarily reverts to normal.

It is vital to have adequate exposure of the internal carotid and control distal to the plaque prior to opening the vessel. The extent of the plaque can be readily palpated with some experience by a moistened finger. There is also a visual cue where the vessel becomes pinker (instead of hard and yellow) and more normal-appearing distal to the extent of the plaque. If high exposure is needed, the posterior belly of the digastric muscle can be cut with impunity, although this is necessary only in a small percentage of cases. For extreme high exposures, the technique of mandibular subluxation for high exposure has been well-described by Simonian et al. (322). In my opinion, it should be rarely needed for routine cases if anatomical principles are followed. We also use a sterile marking pen to draw the proposed arteriotomy line along the vessel, which is helpful in preventing a jagged or curving suture line. When complete exposure is achieved, the final step in preparation for cross-clamping is to ensure that the small spring-loaded Loftus shunt clamp fits snugly around the ICA (see Fig. 3-35).

We then recheck the monitoring system and notify the encephalographer of impending cross-clamping. Once a suitable period of baseline EEG has been recorded, the common carotid is occluded with a large DeBakey vascular clamp and small, straight bulldog clamps or aneurysm clips are used to occlude the ICA and ECA. We always occlude the internal carotid first in the belief that this approach has the lowest risk of embolization associated with clamping. A No. 11 blade is then used to begin the arteriotomy in the common carotid and when the lumen is identified, a Pott's scissors is used to cut straight up along the marked line into the region of the bifurcation and then up into the internal until normal internal carotid is entered. In severely stenotic vessels with friable plaques, the lumen is not always easily discerned and false planes within the lesion are often encountered; great care must be taken to ensure that the back wall of the carotid is not lacerated and that the true lumen is identified prior to attempted shunt insertion.

Changes in the EEG mandate a rapid trial of induced hypertension. If there is no immediate reversal of these changes, an intraluminal shunt is used. The wisdom of shunt use was discussed earlier. Numerous shunt types are available and are a matter of surgeon's familiarity and preference. We have developed and prefer a custom indwelling shunt of our own design (285) (Loftus Carotid Endarterectomy Shunt, Integra Neurocare, Plainsboro, NJ), which is a 15 cm straight silicone tube, supplied in two diameters in the same kit, with tapered ends for easy insertion and a bulb at the proximal end to facilitate anchoring by the Rummel tourniquet. This shunt has a black marker band directly in the center of the shunt, so that cephalad shunt migration can be readily discerned and corrected (see Fig. 3-50). The shunt is first inserted into the CCA and secured by pulling up on the silk ties, a mosquito clamp then holds the rubber sleeve in place to snug the silk around both the vessel and the intraluminal shunt. The shunt tubing is held closed at its midportion with a heavy vascular forceps, then briefly opened to confirm blood flow and evacuate any debris in the shunt tubing. The assistant then uses a microsuction to elucidate the lumen of the internal carotid and the distal end of the shunt tubing is placed at the ICA orifice. After the shunt is again bled flushing any debris from the internal carotid, the bulldog clamp is removed and the shunt is advanced up the internal carotid until the black dot lies in the center of the arteriotomy. The shunt, if properly placed, should slide easily up the internal carotid, and no undue force should be employed, in order to prevent intimal damage and possible dissection (293). The small Javid clamp, or a custom spring clamp specifically designed for the Loftus (or any other) shunt (Loftus Shunt Clamp, Scanlan Instruments, St. Paul, MN) is then used to secure the shunt distally in the internal carotid. Visualization of the dot in the center of the arteriotomy confirms constant correct positioning of the shunt. A hand-held Doppler probe can be applied to the shunt tubing to audibly confirm flow.

With or without the shunt, the plaque is next dissected from the arterial wall with a dissecting instrument, which may be a Freer elevator, a Penfield 4, or the special Scanlan plaque dissector. We hold the wall with a fine vascular pickup and move the instrument from side to side developing a plane first in the lateral wall of the arteriotomy. The plaque is usually readily separated in a primary case and we go approximately halfway around the wall before proceeding to the other side. The plaque is then dissected on the medial side of the common carotid and transected proximally with a Pott's or Church style Metzenbaum scissors. A clean feathering away of the plaque is almost never possible in the common carotid and the goal here is to transect the plaque sharply leaving a smooth transition zone. We sometimes like to pass a right-angle clamp between the plaque and the normal vessel and cut sharply along this clamp blade with the No. 15 knife. (It is important to note that, despite the direction of flow, the proximal endpoint can create a flap and the surgeon should ensure that the common carotid endpoint is adherent.) We then move to the internal carotid where likewise the plaque is dissected first laterally and then medially and then an attempt is made to feather the plaque down smoothly from the internal. Clearly, the ability to establish a clean ICA endpoint improves with greater surgical experience, and the surgeon will use tacking sutures less often as he/she develops the anatomical knowledge and dissection skills for higher ICA exposure in routine cases. However, we find that in some exceptional cases no matter how far up the ICA we go, a shelf of normal intima remains and tacking sutures are required. Often this results from a hurried and over-aggressive ICA dissection from tugging or pulling on the ICA plaque where the actual problem is not residual atheromatous plaque but rather the lifting of normal intima itself (which of course will never taper off).

Attention is finally directed to the final point of plaque attachment at the orifice of the external carotid. The vascular pickup is used to grip across the entire plaque at the external carotid opening and with some traction on the plaque, the external carotid can be everted such that the plaque can be dissected quite far up into that vessel. The eversion of the external and thus optimal plaque removal can be facilitated by "pushing" the distal external proximally with the clamp or forceps. Plaque is often tethered in the external carotid by the clamp and as long as the lumen is held closed with the heavy forceps, this clamp can be removed without untoward bleeding, allowing avulsion of the distal plaque. The clamp must be quickly reapplied to stem the backbleeding that occurs when the plaque is removed from the external. It should be stressed that if plaque removal is inadequate in the external carotid, thrombosis may ensue that can occlude the entire carotid tree with disastrous results. If there is any question of incomplete removal of external plaque, we do not hesitate to extend the arteriotomy up the external carotid itself and close it via a separate suture line.

Following gross plaque removal, we make a careful search for remaining fragments adherent to the arterial wall. Suspect areas are gently stroked with a Kittner "peanut" sponge and every attempt is made to remove all loose fragments in a circumferential fashion, elevating them the complete width of the vessel until they break free at the arteriotomy edge. While it is important to remove all loose fragments, no attempt is made to elevate firmly attached fragments that pose no danger of elevating or breaking off.

Several special aspects of plaque removal need to be considered. The simplest plaques to remove are the soft, friable plaques with intraplaque hemorrhage and thrombus that dissect quite readily and from which fragments are easily removed. The more difficult are the severely stenotic, stony hard plaques in which a plane of dissection at the lateral border of the carotid may be difficult to develop. This situation is analogous to the gross appearance in a case of recurrent carotid stenosis. In several (very rare) of our cases of this type, plaque removal, even in the gentlest fashion, has resulted in areas of thinning where only an adventitial layer is left in the posterior wall of the carotid. We have treated this problem by primary plication of the thin spot with one or two double-armed interrupted stitches of 6-0 Prolene placed in the same fashion as tacking sutures (from the inside out, with the knot outside the vessel). Likewise, we have occasionally encountered an intraluminal thrombus emanating from a congenital web or shelf in the lumen of the vessel (which remains even after endarterectomy), and this has been successfully plicated with a posteriorly placed stitch of double-armed 6-0 Prolene. Finally, in an occasional case where a thin wall looks transparent following declamping, we have reinforced this segment with an encircling buttress of vascular Dacron, sewn together at the top to surround the artery like a pig in a blanket (some call this a "diaper"). We have never seen a carotid blowout postoperatively. In all cases, the goal is to leave as smooth an arteriotomy bed as is possible with minimal areas of denudation or roughness available as sites for thrombus formation.

Attention is then directed to the arterial repair. If desired, the operating microscope can be brought into the field at this point, or in some cases a bit sooner to allow for removal of the small fragments under high magnification. Our personal preference is to continue with $3.5\times$ loupe magnification. As previously mentioned, we use tacking sutures in the distal internal carotid from time to time. Clearly, the need for this decreases with greater surgical experience and with higher dissection up the ICA well beyond the diseased segment. When required, double armed sutures of 6-0 Prolene are placed vertically from the inside of the vessel out, such that they traverse the intimal edge and are tied outside the adventitial layer. Most often, two such sutures are used, placed at the four and eight o'clock positions. The patch, whatever material is employed, is then fashioned, if the surgeon has chosen this option. The patch material (Hemashield in my practice) is placed over the arteriotomy and cut to the exact length of the opening. After removal from the field, the ends are trimmed and tapered to a point with our special Scanlan scissors. Each end of the patch is then anchored to the arteriotomy with double-armed 6-0 Prolene sutures and the needles are left on and secured with rubber-shod clamps. The medial wall suture line is closed first, and a running nonlocking stitch is brought from the ICA anchor to the CCA anchor where it is tied to a free end of the CCA anchor Prolene. At this point, the suture line can be inspected from the inside out. The lateral wall is then closed (with the remaining limb of the ICA anchor stitch) from the ICA to just below the level of the carotid bulb. At this point the second arm of the CCA anchor stitch is used to run up the CCA lateral wall to meet the ICA limb. Small bites are taken just at the arterial edge throughout (being certain, however, that all layers are included), and the suture throws are placed relatively close together to prevent leaks. We also take care that no stray adventitial tags or suture ends are sewn into the lumen where they might induce thrombosis. Several millimeters of unsewn vessel are left on the lateral wall ensuring room to remove the shunt, if one has been used. After the electroencephalographer is again notified, the shunt is double-clamped with two parallel straight mosquitoes, then cut between them and removed in two sections, one from each end. A common error at this point is to mistakenly entangle the suture material in the shunt clamps and thereby hamper smooth shunt removal.

With or without shunt, the arteriotomy is completely closed as follows: All three vessels are first opened and closed sequentially to ensure that backbleeding is present from the ICA, ECA, and CCA. We then re-backbleed the ICA quickly just to be certain that nothing was blown up into the blind sac there. The two stitches are then held taut by the surgeon while the assistant introduces a heparinized saline syringe with blunt needle into the arterial lumen. The vessel is filled with heparinized saline and in this process all air is evacuated from the lumen. As the stitches are drawn up and a surgeon's knot is thrown, the blunt needle is withdrawn allowing no air to enter. Ten more knots are then placed in this most crucial stitch. Declamping is done first from the external carotid, then from the common carotid and finally, at least 10 seconds later, from the ICA. By following this convention, we are assured that all loose debris and remaining microbubbles of air are flushed into the external carotid circulation. Meticulous attention is paid to evacuation of all debris and air prior to opening the internal carotid in every case. However, in the rare case where there is a known external carotid occlusion (although most of these can be reopened at surgery with an ECA endarterectomy), this technique is extremely crucial as there is no external carotid safety valve and all intraluminal contents will be shunted directly into the intracranial circulation.

An alternative method for completing the repair involves removal of the ligature or clip from the superior thyroid artery or external carotid prior to final closure, allowing backbleeding from that vessel to fill the lumen and eliminate the air and debris while the final stitches are placed and tied. This is not my choice simply because I dislike any form of bleeding in the wound.

When the clamps have been removed, we inspect the suture lines for leaks that are customarily controlled with pressure, patience, and surgicel gauze. In occasional cases, a single throw of 6-0 Prolene is necessary to close a persistent arterial hemorrhage. Suture repairs of bleeding points are more likely if a patch graft has been placed. It is almost never necessary to reapply clamps to the artery if the repair has been properly performed. The repair is then lined with surgicel gauze and the three vessels are auscultated with a handheld Doppler to ensure patency. Retractors are removed and hemostasis is confirmed both along the jugular vein and from the surrounding soft tissues. Persistent oozing is often encountered in these patients who have often received large doses of antiplatelet agents in addition to their intraoperative heparin. A final Doppler check is made and the wound is closed in layers. Many vascular surgeons recommend completion duplex ultrasonography at this point to evaluate the status of the repair although we do not do this routinely. The carotid sheath is first closed to provide a barrier against infection, and the platysma is then closed as a separate layer to ensure a good cosmetic result. Either running or interrupted subcuticular stitches may be used to close the skin edges, followed by steri-strips or Dermabond. A Hemovac drain is always used and left inside the carotid sheath to be removed on the first postoperative day. Patients are continued on aspirin following surgery and are discharged in 1 to 2 days. Next-day discharge is feasible and proven safe in many patients who do not have significant medical comorbidities (323).

We manage any postoperative neurological deficit, including TIA alone, with immediate assessment of the technical adequacy of repair. If high-quality color duplex ultrasonography is available, this may allow quick documentation of patency and identify any partially obstructing defects. Angiography is performed if ultrasonography is indeterminate or unavailable. Any occluded carotid postoperation is reexplored and repatched immediately, although since adopting the primary Hemashield patch repair the incidence of postoperative occlusion has been zero.

SPECIAL CONSIDERATIONS

Microsurgical Endarterectomy

Magnified vision and superior lighting have always been essential elements of carotid artery repair. Multiple reports in the neurosurgical literature on microsurgical CEA document excellent morbidity and mortality, equal to or better than the best available published series of conventional surgical technique (295,324,325). Steiger reported 0% morbidity and 2% mortality in a series of 100 consecutive microscopic CEAs (325). The main thrust of this article was TCD and EEG monitoring. However, the microsurgical technique was mentioned as a surgical improvement as well. Spetzler et al. made recommendations for a careful approach to risk reduction in CEA that included microsurgical endarterectomy. They emphasized that the operative microscope was brought into the field not throughout the case but rather after gross removal of the plaque and just prior to final cleaning of the vessel in preparation for arterial repair. These authors emphasized the value of the microscope in performing a finer and less stenotic arterial repair as well as providing the necessary vision and illumination to facilitate removal of all retained fragments and debris. Morbidity and mortality in this series was 1.5% (295). Findlay and Lougheed, reporting a series of 60 patients with a 2% morbidity and mortality (324), outlined a somewhat different technique. These authors brought the microscope into the field following dissection of the arterial tree but prior to arterial cross-clamping and performance of the arteriotomy itself.

No controlled or randomized series of microsurgical endarterectomy is available. Nonetheless, the excellent results from these three series imply that microsurgical endarterectomy may become increasingly accepted.

Bilateral Carotid Endarterectomy

Bilateral symptomatic carotid lesions are unusual, but occasionally patients may present with stereotypic TIAs referable to both carotid circulations. The surgeon's dilemma then becomes which procedure should be performed first. It has been my preference to operate first on the side with the most recent or crescendo TIAs. On several occasions, however, I have opted to operate first on the side with a preocclusive lesion, with the idea that reconstruction of the opposite carotid first would lead to thrombosis of a 99% lesion once collateral circulation was increased.

For symptomatic disease with an asymptomatic contralateral lesion that meets the ACAS criteria, we choose staged procedures with repair of the symptomatic side first. For bilateral asymptomatic disease that meets the ACAS criteria, we repair the highest grade stenosis side first. Basically, the policy in my practice is to repair the more dangerous lesion first since there is a small possibility that a second side cannot be done because of cranial/cervical nerve issues (see below).

Bilateral CEA runs the risk of not only extreme swings of blood pressure from concurrent denervation of both carotid sinuses (326), but also the risk of bilateral cranial nerve injury. For this reason, when bilateral CEA is required in my patients, I stage these procedures six weeks apart whenever possible and have the patient examined by an otolaryngologist to ensure that no occult cranial nerve or vocal cord dysfunction is present prior to the second procedure. Unilateral nerve dysfunction in the cervical region is troublesome but a bilateral one can be disabling. I have, on several occasions, deferred second side surgery and maintained the patient on medical therapy when an occult vocal cord paralysis was diagnosed. I have also performed bilateral CEAs as soon as 72 hours apart when the patient had crescendo TIAs from both vessels and needed to be maintained on heparin.

Complete Occlusion

My surgical technique for complete CCA/ICA occlusion (see Figs. 4-1 to 4-3) involves opening (or reopening) of the CCA and ICA once all vessels have been controlled. Thrombus is usually seen at the carotid bulb and extending into the distal ICA; in my experience, the ECA usually is patent. Removal of thrombus and associated

ICA plaque may establish backbleeding; if not, the ICA can be explored with a No. 8 feeding tube cut to 15 cm length and attached to a 10 cc syringe. The tube is advanced into the ICA and the syringe is drawn back to establish suction, which often will pull down the distal thrombus as the tubing is withdrawn. If this fails, Fogarty catheters are passed into the ICA but the associated risk of creating a carotid-cavernous fistula with these devices should be kept in mind. If backbleeding cannot be established, I ligate the distal and proximal ICA stump and perform a CCA/ECA endarterectomy and roof patch repair.

Acute Stroke

Surgical technique for acute stroke patients differs little from standard CEA (147,159,327, 328). I will operate on stroke patients if they have a normal level of consciousness and no hemorrhage or mass effect on head CT scan. Some patients may be fully heparinized, and as mentioned above we no longer recommend cessation of heparin six hours prior to surgery as we had done previously. The question of insensitive EEG monitoring in acute stroke exists, leading some to recommend empirical shunt placement, although I do not follow this practice. Intraoperative and perioperative hypertension must be strictly controlled in the setting of a dysautoregulated cerebral hemisphere (329).

POSTOPERATIVE CONSIDERATIONS

Following CEA, the patient is awakened in the operating room and does not leave until a screening neurologic examination has been performed. A skilled anesthestist and rapid emergence from anesthesia is crucial; few things are more troublesome than a patient who remains deeply anesthetized or who has been overtreated with paralytic agents and who thus cannot be examined for 30 to 60 anxious minutes. The superficial temporal artery (STA) pulse, which was checked preoperatively, is palpated again on the operative side. I anticipate that all carotid patients will be neurologically intact at the conclusion of the procedure. We examine them carefully for grip strength, function of the hypoglossal nerve, and function of the marginal mandibular branch of the facial nerve (by asking them to smile). Patients who are neurologically unstable preoperatively or who have had a preexistent stroke, may sometimes have some decreased grip strength for the first several postoperative hours. Typically, this is a transient phenomenon that occasionally responds to a slight increase of blood pressure and almost always resolves spontaneously. However, the process of waiting for this to resolve is nerve wracking for the surgeon. I take comfort in the fact that I have tested the artery with the intraoperative Doppler following the repair and immediately prior to closing the neck. Patients who were normal preoperatively and who awaken with a new postoperative deficit, however, or stroke patients who do not appear to be making steady progress over the first several hours, have a duplex scan (if readily available), or are taken immediately to the angiographic suite to confirm patency of the vessel. If there is any question of inadequate technical repair or a postoperative occlusion, I return to surgery for reexploration of the wound.

I have not adopted the policy of exploring the wound without radiographic confirmation of technical error in patients who awaken with a neurologic deficit. I prefer to obtain a good snapshot of the anatomy and areas of technical difficulty prior to reexploring the vessel. Most patients who undergo angiography do not, in fact, have an identified technical error, and most go on to make a reasonable recovery from what is assumed to be a transient ischemic deficit. My overall perioperative stroke rate in patients (including all classes of preoperative risk) has been gratifyingly less than 2%.

I monitor all patients in the recovery room for an hour or so and then transfer them to the intensive care unit for overnight observation prior to return to the dedicated stroke unit. I choose ICU management of the patients primarily for control of blood pressure, and prevention of the risk of MI. It is my goal to support with pressors a systolic blood pressure (SBP) below 100 mmHg, and to use antihypertensive therapy if the SBP exceeds 160 mmHg. It is especially important to control hypertension in patients who have had reopening of a tight stenosis, since the ipsilateral cerebral hemisphere is most likely dysautoregulated and hypertension may predispose these patients to intracerebral hemorrhage (329). Following transfer to the floor the following day, the Hemovac is removed and the patient is mobilized. They are discharged on the third hospital day essentially without exception. Since the wound is customarily closed with subcuticular stitches, there is no need for suture removal.

My long term follow-up of carotid patients involves a visit at six weeks and another at three months. We routinely perform a postoperative duplex examination at three months and then at six month intervals thereafter to follow both the operated and the silent side. Patients are maintained on aspirin, 325 mg daily for the rest of their lives.

COMPLICATIONS OF CEA

It is generally recognized that patients with cerebrovascular disease severe enough to warrant carotid artery surgery often have serious associated medical conditions, and that the surgical morbidity and mortality risks in such patients are directly related to the degree of these complicating systemic factors. Several authors have demonstrated that perioperative risks of 1% in patients without associated medical or angiographic risk factors increase to at least 7% in individuals with such predisposing medical conditions as angina pectoris, recent MI, congestive heart failure, severe hypertension, chronic obstructive pulmonary disease, or obesity (330,331). Nonetheless, patients with classical carotid symptoms who are consequently at high risk for embolic stroke may still benefit from surgical therapy, and all precautions must be taken to avoid aggravating underlying disease.

The NASCET experience with medical complications has been elegantly analyzed as a separate manuscript (332). Most complications were cardiovascular and occurred in patients with known risk factors, and most completely resolved without sequelae.

The endovascular community makes a strong argument that "high-risk" carotid surgery should be deferred in favor of carotid stenting, and cites the SAPPHIRE industry-funded trial to support this (141). The precise definition of high risk varies by surgeon and surgical experience, but is generally accepted to include medical comorbidities, recurrent disease, anatomical variants (long or high lesions), radiation-induced atherosclerosis, and in some opinions, contralateral occlusion. Clearly, this is a controversial subject. Two recent large, quality studies showed no difference at all in stroke rate between patients with one or more of these common risk factors and "no risk factor" patients (333,334). Another excellent study from UCLA shows that CEA in radiation atherosclerosis is safe, durable, and confers no greater risk than in routine (nonirradiated) patients (335).

Endovascular specialists also champion protected carotid stenting as a benign alternative to CEA in elderly patients. Two contemporary studies dispute and to some extent refute this logic. Kastrup et al. showed a significantly higher 30-day stroke rate in CAS patients than in CEA patients (age >75 years) (336). Similarly, in the lead-in (credentialing) phase of CREST, alarmingly high complication rates for CAS increased linearly with age (stroke/death 1.3%, age 60–69; 5.3%, age 70–79; 12.1% age >80) (337). It is also clear that treatment for elderly patients is warranted; the NASCET subgroup analysis shows that elderly patients with symptomatic 50% to 99% stenosis benefited more from CEA than younger patients in the prevention of ipsilateral ischemic stroke (338).

The SAPPHIRE data are provocative, but cannot be accepted with the same level of evidence as the government-funded NASCET or ACAS trials. Large numbers of patients (407) were treated (stented) outside of the randomization process, and no outcome data are given for this group. Only seven patients were operated outside of the randomized group. If these nonrandomized CAS patients were at a higher risk than the overall group, and had a higher complication rate, then the trial would be biased against CEA. Likewise, many of the SAPPHIRE-treated patients were asymptomatic, and their comorbidities were severe enough that by most guidelines documents they would have been considered unsuitable for treatment. In the symptomatic SAPPHIRE group, where patients were appropriate for treatment, there was no difference between surgery and stenting for this high-risk group.

The complications of CEA can be divided into three major groups, those associated with perioperative medical and anesthetic nonneurologic events; those involving vascular events in the territory of the operated carotid; and those related to local-wound problems.

The major nonneurologic perioperative complication of carotid surgery is MI, the incidence of which is from 1% to 4% (339–342) in carotid procedures. As Sundt et al. have demonstrated, the risk of carotid surgery is markedly increased in patients with definite histories of cardiac disease (330). Yeager et al. also showed that diabetes mellitus was a significant risk factor for perioperative MI in their series of 249 procedures (342), and Riles et al. showed that the use of vasopressors in CEA patients was associated with a fourfold rise (2.0% to 8.1%) in the incidence of postoperative MI (340).

Complications referable to the vascular territory of the operated carotid artery include devastating embolic, ischemic, and/or hemorrhagic strokes, and, rarely, postoperative TIAs. Postoperative stroke rates, although generally decreasing with advances in surgical and anesthetic skills, vary from Sundt's figure of 0.6% embolic stroke to a rate of 14.5% in one community hospital series (343). It is generally accepted that embolic stroke rates can be reduced by the gentlest possible dissection of the carotid, and that thrombosis of the operated carotid is often a reflection of technical error, whether from dissection of a distal intimal flap or stenosis in the arteriotomy suture line (331). Postoperative hypotension, the consequence of carotid baroreceptor dysfunction (344,345) has been shown to be associated with an increased incidence of complications (344,346), and may contribute to ischemic neurologic deficits. The etiology of the commonly observed postoperative hypertension and its effect on hemorrhagic stroke is less well understood (344). There is good evidence, however, that clinically elevated preoperative blood pressure is the major contributing factor in this problem, and in one study the incidences of both postoperative neurologic deficit and operative death were significantly increased in the patient group manifesting postoperative hypertension (347).

Postendarterectomy hemorrhagic complications are probably multifactorial. Hyperperfusion related to revascularization of a severe stenosis and systemic essential hypertension plays a predominant role (329). Several groups have confirmed the risk profile of younger patients with tight carotid stenosis and hypertension, and emphasize the postoperative prodrome of severe headache, in predicting post-CEA intracerebral hemorrhage (329,348). Hosoda et al. (349) present evidence that impaired cerebral vasoreactivity measured with acetazolamide-challenge SPECT can predict postoperative hyperperfusion; however, most hyperperfusion does not result in frank intracerebral hemorrhage (ICH) (349). Massive fatal ICH has been reported following carotid stenting as well, again in a patient with tight stenosis, although normotensive at baseline (350).

The use of anticoagulants or perhaps antiplatelet-aggregating medications can be implicated in some cases of perioperative hemorrhage, and they should be used with caution and an awareness of the increase in risk. Postoperative TIAs are disturbing in that they may represent acute carotid occlusion requiring surgical intervention. Nonocclusive TIAs, however, have been successfully managed with anticoagulation (330).

Rapid postoperative onset of neurological deficit elicits various responses from surgeons. Some advocate immediate return to surgery for reopening of the (presumably occluded) artery. In my experience most such cases, especially with patch grafting, are patent when investigated, and I now prefer to manage any postoperative neurologic deficit, including TIA alone, with immediate duplex scanning if available. If the vessel is occluded by duplex, the patient is explored. If the vessel appears patent, and the deficit is more than fleeting, we proceed to angiography, looking for a technical inadequacy that might warrant heparinization, or for intracranial embolic problems that might benefit from supraselective catheterization and thrombolysis.

Radak et al. have analyzed causes of perioperative stroke in 2250 cases. As most experienced surgeons would intuitively suspect, their data show that intraoperative stroke (patient awakens with deficit) is usually from an uncorrectable cause, whereas postoperative stroke is most likely from technical error or technique-associated thrombosis or mural thrombus (351).

Problems related to the wound constitute the final group of carotid surgical complications. Injuries to local cranial nerves, including the marginal mandibular, hypoglossal, superior laryngeal, and recurrent laryngeal nerves are among the most common of these complications, and in one prospective series such an injury was found in 12.5% of patients (352). The majority of these injuries were subclinical or mild and recovered spontaneously, and were attributed to retraction rather than transection injury. The incidence of hemorrhage from the carotid suture line is low, much less than 1% in two major series (330,341) despite the use of intraoperative anticoagulants (353). Such hemorrhage can, however, be catastrophic with tracheal obstruction and can lead to false aneurysm formation (354). Wound infections, usually with *Staphylococcus* species, occasionally have been reported and may rarely contribute to the genesis of a false aneurysm (355).

Most complications from CEA occur within 24 hours of surgery (323). Early discharge is appropriate and increasingly favored in light of this. Sheehan et al. analyzed CEA complications and found that 95% of patients with either new neurological deficits or neck hematomas (either of which could require reoperation) presented within eight hours postoperation (356). They used these data to support a policy of same-evening discharge following CEA for selected cases, a policy which I personally have not adopted.

ENDOVASCULAR TREATMENT OF CAROTID STENOSIS

Endovascular techniques including angioplasty and stenting are alternatives to CEA for the treatment of carotid occlusive disease. At the present time, I feel that endovascular techniques are indicated for patients who are not candidates for conventional open reconstruction. The available literature supports this. This may include patients with extremely high lesions and patients with medical contraindications to GA (pulmonary or cardiac). Some experts feel that recurrent carotid stenosis and patients with contralateral carotid occlusion are better treated by endovascular techniques, as mentioned above. The SAPPHIRE trial data show that clinical outcomes are no different for surgery (CEA) or protected stenting (CAS) for "high-risk" carotid lesions.

Given the increasingly widespread availability of stenting, we must then ask ourselves whether there is an outcome-based reason to choose endovascular over surgical treatment.

If we look at the surgical results from randomized cooperative trials, we see that the complication rates are gratifyingly quite low. In the ACAS trial, the perioperative stroke and death rate was 2.3%. In the VAAST trial, the 30-day mortality was 1.9%, all referable to MI. The perioperative stroke rate was 2.4%. The nerve injury rate was 3.8% and the rate of nonfatal MI was likewise 1.9%.

In evaluating the results of symptomatic cooperative trials, we look first at the NASCET Trial (69) where the 30-day mortality was 0.6%. The perioperative major stroke and death rate was 2.1%. The all-stroke rate was 5.5%. The nerve injury rate, evaluated by independent examiners, was 7.6%, the wound hematoma rate was 5.5%, and the MI rate was 0.9%. In the ECST symptomatic cooperative trial (71), it is very-difficult to tease out the major stroke or death rate because the data are presented in different manuscripts. However, it appears to be quite variable depending on the stratification of percent stenosis being considered. In the 0 to 29% surgery group, the major death or stroke rate was 2.3%. In the 30% to 49% group it was 8%. In the 50% to 69% group, it was 7.9%, and in the 70% to 99% group, it was 3.7%. In the VASST (74), the 30-day mortality was 3.3%, the perioperative stroke rate was 2.2%, the nerve injury rate was 5%, the wound hematoma rate was 5%, and the MI rate was 2%.

If we look at the results, cooperative trials customarily represent fixed observation points and evaluation by nonbiased observers. Randomized trial data are often felt to be the most valid and the highest level of evidence data that we have available to make therapeutic judgements. If we look at the published results of individual skilled carotid surgeons (see below), we come up with data that shed a bit more of a favorable light on carotid reconstruction. It is to be recalled, nonetheless, that essentially all the major cooperative trials demonstrated that carotid artery surgery was superior to medical therapy despite their higher complication rates as compared to the results of individual surgeons.

Returning to the individual surgeon's published results category, the data published by Spetzler (295) for carotid microsurgery show that in 200 cases, the all-stroke rate was 1%, the mortality was 0.5%, the wound hematoma rate was 1.5%, and the nerve injury rate was 5%. The data presented by Findlay (324) in carotid microsurgery document an all-stroke rate of 1.7%, a wound hematoma rate of 3.3%, and a nerve injury rate of 5.1%. The data presented by Steiger (325), again considering carotid microsurgery, document a perioperative stroke rate of zero, an MI rate of 2%, a mortality of 2%, and a nerve injury rate of 2%. The data presented by Harbaugh (180) employing RA with loupe-magnified carotid reconstruction shows an all-stroke rate of 2.5% with an ipsilateral rate of 1.3%, and a major stroke rate of 0.9%. Harbaugh's MI rate is 1.3%. The wound hematoma rate is 2.1%, and the nerve injury rate is 3%. Finally, my own data representing conventional loupe-magnified carotid reconstruction, under GA, with Hemashield patch angioplasty in the second half of the series, show an all-stroke rate of 1.8% with a major stroke rate of 0.72%. My mortality rate is 0.72% and my wound hematoma rate is 0.4% (156,161).

If we look then at the data from leading surgeons published on an individual basis with their own observations of complications, we find that the all-stroke rate is customarily less than 2.6%, the nerve injury rate is less than 5.1%, the mortality is less than 2%, and the wound hematoma rate varies between a low of 0.35% to a high of 3.35%.

Let us then consider the published and reported results for carotid stenting, with and without distal protective devices. Several studies have demonstrated acceptable morbidity and mortality data for the use of carotid angioplasty and stenting in carotid stenosis. Diethrich et al. (357) reported 110 patients (117 vessels), 79 of whom were asymptomatic and 31 of whom were symptomatic with stenosis greater than or equal to 70%. Two major and five minor neurological events resulted from the procedure, together representing 6.4% of the study population. TIAs were reported in five patients, with a 1.8% mortality. Asymptomatic occlusion occurred in 1.8% and 2.7% ultimately required endarterectomy for failure or restenosis. Theron et al. reported stenting patients with primary stenosis (358). This paper discusses a protection scheme in about half the patients with distal balloon protection being employed during the stenting procedure. Two-hundred and fifty-nine patients were treated of which 136 underwent cerebral protection and 123 did not. In the unprotected cases, the rate of carotid dissection was 5% and the rate of embolization was 8%. In the protected cases, no dissection is reported and the embolization rate is 1%. Some of these patients were not stented but merely had angioplasty. In these authors' experience, stenting reduced the restenosis rate from 16% to 4% and the authors' conclusion was that all patients undergoing endovascular carotid treatment should be stented and should be treated with cerebral protective strategies during the stenting process.

Yadav et al. (359) reported 126 treated arteries, all stented. There were seven minor strokes, two major strokes, and one death in this series. The stroke and death rate was 7.9% with an ipsilateral major stroke risk of 1.6%. The restenosis rate was quoted at 4.9%; all of these patients were asymptomatic. Yadav concluded that it was feasible to stent high-risk carotid patients who were not considered to be surgical candidates. Guterman and Hopkins (360) relayed their experience with 96 high medical risk patients with unstable angina or restenosis after endarterectomy. Patients with long stenotic segments or high-carotid bifurcations were also included. Angioplasty and stent placement was undertaken in 62 patients, with the remainder receiving angioplasty alone. Two deaths of cardiac origin, two minor strokes, and no major complications were reported. The experience of Rosenwasser and Shanno (361) with 47 patients treated with angioplasty (45 of whom also had stents placed) revealed one major stroke five days postoperatively and one "cold foot" that resolved with heparin therapy. Sixty-three percent required temporary pacing during inflation (29/47 patients). Their indications for endovascular treatment of carotid occlusive disease were radiation-induced stenosis, recurrent stenosis, medically unstable patients (with cardiac or pulmonary risk factors), and lesions at C1-2 or long lesions extending into the petrous segment.

Interesting data are reported by Lanzino et al. (362) regarding recurrent carotid stenosis. Lanzino and collaborators treated 25 arteries for recurrent stenosis with percutaneous angioplasty alone in 7 and placement of a stent in 18. There were no major neurological or cardiac events. Complications were limited to one TIA and one femoral pseudoaneurysm. Lanzino et al. demonstrated that 60% of angioplasty- alone patients restenosed and only one stent patient restenosed. Accordingly, their recommendation was first that the stenting procedure without protective strategies was safe for recurrent carotid stenosis and that stenting was far superior to angioplasty alone in the treatment of restenotic carotid disease.

Randomized trial data are now available for CAS. In the first such study by Naylor et al. (363) in the United Kingdom randomized trial of angioplasty/stenting versus carotid surgery, 23 patients were randomized who had greater than or equal to 70% carotid stenosis. Seventeen of these patients were treated, 10 of whom had carotid surgery with no complications. Seven patients underwent either angioplasty or stent and five of these patients had a stroke. This trial was prematurely stopped because of an extremely negative outcome in the endovascular side and has been reported as strong evidence to suggest that carotid surgery is superior to endovascular carotid treatment. The Schneider wallstent trial (364) was also stopped prematurely, because a futility analysis showed that there was no possibility that CAS would be equal to or superior to CEA. Morbidity figures in this trial for CAS were fourfold the surgical figures.

The SAPPHIRE (141) trial randomized "high-risk" carotid stenosis patients, both asymptomatic and symptomatic, to CAS or CEA. Both techniques were effective, with statistically equal risk, in the treatment of symptomatic patients. For asymptomatic patients, there was a trend (p = NS) to lower risk with CAS. Questions have been raised, however, whether high-risk asymptomatic patients should be treated at all, since AHA guidelines have specified that surgical treatment is inappropriate for these patients. The only true answer to this question would be a study of CAS versus medical therapy in this group. No such study exists at present.

As this book is written, patient entry and randomization continues for the NIH funded Carotid Revascularization Endarterectomy versus Stent Trial (CREST) of CEA versus CAS in non-high-risk patients. CREST, and other similar trials in Europe and in Japan will hopefully provide a definitive level 1 evidence basis for therapeutic decision making.

Nonatheromatous lesions, such as fibromuscular dysplasia, have also been studied with endovascular treatment. Hasso et al. (365) report three cases, all of which were symptomatic, that were treated with angioplasty alone in which no complications were evident. This is an extremely small series but it represents essentially the only experience in the literature regarding the endovascular treatment of fibromuscular dysplasia.

If endovascular treatment is to be considered we should likewise ask the question "which lesions are there which the surgeon does not want to operate on?" This brings to my mind the question of what constitutes a high-risk carotid operation. I would put high-risk patients in several categories. The first consists of patients who have predictably difficult operations. The second consists of patients who are at a high risk for medical complications. The third consists of patients who are at a high risk for intraoperative ischemia, and the fourth consists of patients who, for anatomical or other reasons, are at high risk for postoperative occlusion and/or stroke.

Considering the first category, predictably difficult operations would include anatomical variants such as a medially directed ICA, a long and high carotid plaque, a high carotid bifurcation, or other anatomical anomalies such as cervical carotid aneurysm that would render an operation significantly more difficult. Predictably difficult operations also include carotid reoperation, operation upon carotids that have been previously irradiated for other reasons, and cases in which distal exposure will be extremely high, in the region of C1 or C2 on a lateral angiogram.

In the second category, patients at high risk for medical complication, I would include patients with recent MI, patients with unstable angina, diabetic patients (who in my experience are at high risk for postoperative occlusion), patients with severe pulmonary disease rendering GA a major risk, and patients who require preoperative anticoagulation.

In the third category, those at high risk for intraoperative ischemia, I would include patients with contralateral occlusion, based on the NASCET findings, although in my personal experience this does not appreciably increase the risk. Patients who will have difficult or impossible shunt placement have a high risk for intraoperative ischemia if a shunt is required. This includes patients who have a right-angle bend distal to the carotid plaque and in whom this bend cannot be straightened out through operative exposure, or patients who have a large cervical aneurysm that precludes placement of a shunt. High risk for intraoperative ischemia also includes patients with difficult cervical carotid exposures, patients who are neurologically unstable with a fluctuating deficit, and patients who have a propagating thrombus in the cervical carotid artery distal to an area of high-grade stenosis but who continue to have antegrade flow beyond the region of the thrombus.

Patients at high risk for postoperative occlusion and/or stroke include the following categories. Diabetic patients, in my experience, have a higher risk than normal for a postoperative occlusion, patients who experience postoperative hypotension seem to have a higher risk for carotid occlusion, patients in whom a repair is done high up in the ICA with consequent narrowing of the internal carotid are at high risk for occlusion and patients who are hypertensive who experience dysautoregulation type headache following reconstruction of a tight stenosis are at high risk for postoperative intracerebral hemorrhage. In my experience, most of these complications, with the exception of ICH, are avoided by universal use of the Hemashield patch graft and the luxuriant large lumen that it affords.

I believe that protected stenting, performed by qualified and credentialed operators, has a major role in selected carotid disease. Cases I might send for stenting include cases of carotid dissection, which we previously treated with anticoagulation alone, and which may well be managed by a careful cannulation of the vessel and crossing of the lesion followed by placement of a stent. This, in my mind, represents a very significant advance over any surgical treatment or over anticoagulation alone as a therapeutic strategy. Cases with high cervical carotid aneurysms, beyond the reach of the surgeon, are well treated by stenting across the mouth of the lesion. Cases in which extreme high exposures are required at the base of the skull may well be better treated by stenting than by surgical exposure particularly when one considers the risk of cranial nerve injury. Patients with symptomatic cervical carotid plaques, who are medically unstable or with recent MI, are probably better served when treated with endovascular treatment than with surgery, which entails an increased risk from GA. Finally, cases of fibromuscular dysplasia, as discussed above, which I customarily do not treat with surgery, may well be rational cases for a protected stenting approach.

In conclusion, it is my opinion that the endovascular versus surgical debate for carotid artery therapy and/or asymptomatic patients will continue for certainly the next 5 to 10 years, and most likely both treatments will ultimately enjoy some degree of acceptance. I would reiterate that at the present time only carotid artery surgery is proven by level 1 evidence to be superior to medical therapy and endovascular treatment stands where we stood with carotid artery surgery approximately 15 years ago, leaving us with feasibility and registry studies primarily, with some randomized trials available, but as yet none which demonstrate equivalence or superiority to CEA.

REFERENCES

1. Thompson J. The development of carotid artery surgery. Arch Surg 1973; 107:643–648.
2. Abernathy J. Surgical Observations. London: Longman and Rees, 1804.
3. Cooper A. Account of the first successful operation performed on the common carotid artery for aneurysm in the year 1808 with the postmortem examination in the year 1821. Guy Hosp Rep 1836; 1:53.
4. Carrea R, Molins M, Murphy G. Surgical treatment of spontaneous thrombosis of the internal carotid artery in the neck: carotid-carotideal anastomosis, report of a case. Acta Neurol Lat Am 1955; 1:71–78.
5. Wylie E, Kerr E, Davies O. Experimental and clinical experiences with the use of fascia lata applied as a graft after thromboendarterectomy and aneurysmorrhaphy. Surg Gynecol Obstet 1951; 93:257–272.
6. Thompson JE. The evolution of surgery for the treatment and prevention of stroke. The Willis Lecture. Stroke 1996; 27:1427–1434.
7. DeBakey M. Successful carotid endarterectomy for cerebrovascular insufficiency. Nineteen year follow up. J Am Med Assoc 1975; 233:1083–1085.
8. Eastcott H, Pickering G, Rob CG. Reconstruction of internal carotid artery in a patient with intermittent attacks of hemiplegia. Lancet 1954; 2:944–946.
9. Loftus CM. Carotid Endarterectomy: Principles and Technique. St. Louis: Quality Medical Publishing, 1995.
10. Executive Committee for the Asymptomatic Carotid Atheroselerosis Study. Endarterectomy for asymptomatic carotid stenosis. J Am Med Assoc 1995; 273:1421–1428.
11. MRC Asymptomatic Carotid Surgery Trial. Prevention of disabling and fatal strokes by successful carotid endarterectomy in patients without recent neurological symptoms: randomised controlled trial. Lancet 2004; 363:1491–1502.
12. Cooperman M, Martin E, Evans W. Significance of asymptomatic carotid bruits. Arch Surg 1978; 113:1339–1340.
13. Thompson J, Patman R, Talkington C. Asymptomatic carotid bruit. Longterm outcome of patients having endarterectomy compared to unoperated controls. Ann Surg 1978; 188:308–315.
14. Heyman A, et al. Risk of stroke in asymptomatic persons with cervical arterial bruits. A population study in Evans County, Georgia. N Engl J Med 1980; 302:838–841.
15. Wolf P, Kannel W, Sorlie P. Asymptomatic carotid bruit and risk of stroke. The Framingham study. J Am Med Assoc 1981; 245:1442–1445.

16. Norris JW, Zhu CZ. Silent stroke and carotid stenosis. Stroke 1992; 23:483–485.
17. Archie J, Feldtman R. Critical stenosis of the internal carotid artery. Surgery 1981; 89:67–72.
18. Ojemann RG, et al. Surgical treatment of extracranial carotid occlusive disease. Clin Neurosurg 1975; 22:214–263.
19. Roederer GO, et al. The natural history of carotid arterial disease in asymptomatic patients with cervical bruits. Stroke 1984; 15:605–613.
20. Chambers B, Norris J. Outcome in patients with asymptomatic neck bruits. N Engl J Med 1986; 315:860–865.
21. Norris JW, et al. Vascular risks of asymptomatic carotid stenosis. Stroke 1991; 22:1485–1490.
22. Corman L. The preoperative patient with an asymptomatic carotid bruit. Med Clin North Am 1979; 63:1335–1340.
23. Fields W. The asymptomatic carotid bruit—operate or not? Stroke 1978; 9:269–271.
24. Mohr JP. Asymptomatic carotid artery disease. Stroke 1982; 13:431–433.
25. Yatsu FM, Hart RG. Asymptomatic carotid bruit amd stenosis: a reappraisal. Stroke 1983; 14:301–304.
26. Halliday AW. The asymptomatic carotid surgery trial (ACST) rationale and design. Eur J Vasc Surg 1994; 8:703–710.
27. CASANOVA Study Group. Carotid surgery versus medical therapy in asymptomatic carotid stenosis. Stroke 1991; 22:1229–1233.
28. Mayo Asymptomatic Carotid Endarterectomy Study Groups. Results of a randomized controlled trial of carotid endarterectomy for asymptomatic carotid stenosis. Mayo Clin Proc 1992; 67:513–518.
29. Hobson RW, et al. Efficacy of carotid endarterectomy for asymptomatic carotid stenosis. New Engl J Med 1993; 328:221–227.
30. Rockman CB, et al. Carotid endarterectomy in female patients: are the concerns of the Asymptomatic Carotid Atherosclerosis Study valid? J Vasc Surg 2001; 33(2): 236–241.
31. Akbari C, et al. Gender and carotid endarterectomy: does it matter? J Vasc Surg 2000; 31(6): 1103–1109.
32. Biller J, et al. Guidelines for carotid endarterectomy. Stroke 1998; 29:554–562.
33. Durward Q, Ferguson G, Barr H. The natural history of asymptomatic carotid bifurcation plaques. Stroke 1982; 13:459–464.
34. Humphries A, Young J, Santilli P. Unoperated asymptomatic significant internal carotid artery stenosis: a review of 182 cases. Surgery 1976; 80:695– 698.
35. Johnson N, Bumham S, Flanigan D. Carotid endarterectomy: as follow-up study of the contralateral non-operated carotid artery. Ann Surg 1978; 188:748–752.
36. Levin S, Sondheimer F. Stenosis of the contralateral asymptomatic carotid artery—to operate or not? Vasc Surg 1973; 7:3–13.
37. Levin S, Sondheimer F, Levin J. The contralateral diseased but asymptomatic carotid artery—to operate or not? Am J Surg 1980; 140:203–205.
38. Podore P, et al. Asymptomatic contralateral carotid artery stenosis: a five-year follow-up study following carotid endarterectomy. Surgery 1980; 88:748–752.
39. Lefrak E, Guinn G. Prophylactic carotid artery surgery in patients requiring a second operation. South Med J 1974; 67:185–189.
40. Treiman R, Foran R, Shore E. Carotid bruit. Significance in patients undergoing an abdominal aortic operation. Arch Surg 1973; 106:803–805.
41. Treiman R, Foran R, Cohen J. Carotid bruit. A follow-up report on its significance in patients undergoing an abdominal aortic operation. Arch Surg 1979; 114:1138–1140.
42. Evans W, Cooperman M. The significance of asymptomatic unilateral carotid bruits in preoperative patients. Surgery 1978; 83:521–522.
43. Carney W, Stewart W, DePinto D. Carotid bruit as a risk factor in aortoiliac reconstruction. Surgery 1977; 81:567–570.
44. Barnes R, Liebman P, Marszalek P. The natural history of asymptomatic carotid disease in patients undergoing cardiovascular surgery. Surgery 1981; 90:1075–1083.
45. Barnes R, Marszalek P. Asymptomatic carotid disease in the cardiovascular surgical patient: is prophylactic endarterectomy necessary? Stroke 1981; 12:497–500.
46. Breslau P, Fell G, Ivey T. Carotid arterial disease in patients undergoing coronary bypass operations. J Thor Cardiovasc Surg 1981; 82:765–767.
47. Turnipseed W, Berkoff H, Belzer F. Postoperative stroke in cardiac and peripheral vascular disease. Ann Surg 1980; 192:365–368.

48. Ropper A, Wechsler L, Wilson L. Carotid bruit and risk of stroke in elective surgery. N Engl J Med 1982; 307:1388–1390.
49. Martin W, Hashimoto S. Stroke in coronary bypass surgery. Can J Neurol Sci 1982; 9:21–26.
50. Furlan A, Craciun A. Risk of stroke during coronary artery bypass graft surgery in patients with internal carotid artery disease documented by angiography. Stroke 1985; 16:797–799.
51. Hollenhorst R. Significance of bright plaques in the retinal arterioles. J Am Med Assoc 1961; 178:123–129.
52. David N, Klintworth G, Friedberg S. Fatal atheromatous cerebral embolism associated with bright plaques in the retinal arterioles: report of a case. Neurology 1963; 13:708–713.
53. Balla JL Howat ML, Walton JN. Cholesterol emboli in retinal arteries. J Neurol Neurosurg Psychiat 1964; 27:144–148.
54. Russell RW. Atheromatous retinal embolism. Lancet 1963; 2:1354–1356.
55. Russell RW. The source of retinal emboli. Lancet 1968; 2:789–792.
56. Pfaffenbach DD, Hollenhorst RW. Morbidity and survivorship of patients with embolic cholesterol crystals in the ocular fundus. Am J Ophth 1973; 75:66–72.
57. Bruno A, et al. Concomitants of asymptomatic retinal cholesterol emboli. Stroke 1992; 23:900–902.
58. Beebe HG, et al. Assessing risk associated with carotid endarterectomy. Stroke 1989; 20:314–315.
59. American College of Physicians. Indications for carotid endarterectomy. Ann Intern Med 1989; 111:675–677.
60. Acheson J, Hutchinson E. Observations on the natural history of transient cerebral ischemia. Lancet 1964; 2:871.
61. Baker R, Ramseyer J, Schwartz W. Prognosis in patients with transient cerebral ischemic attacks. Neurology 1968; 18:1157–1165.
62. Whisnant J, Matsumoto N, Elveback L. Transient cerebral ischemic attacks in a community: Rochester, Minnesota 1955 through 1969. Mayo Clin Proc 1973; 48:844–848.
63. Whisnant J. Epidemiology of stroke: emphasis on transient cerebral ischemic attacks and hypertension. Stroke 1974; 5:68–70.
64. Whisnant J, Cartlidge N, Elveback L. Carotid and vertebro-basilar transient ischemic attacks: effect of anticoagulants, hypertension, and cardiac disorders on survivat and stroke occurrence—a population study. Ann Neurol 1978; 3:107– 115.
65. Fields W, Lemak N, Frankowski R. Controlled trial of aspirin in cerebral ischemia. Stroke 1977; 8:301–314.
66. Canadian Cooperative Study Group. A randomized trial of aspirin and sulfinpyrazone in threatened stroke. N Engl J Med 1978; 299:53–59.
67. American-Canadian Cooperative Study Group. Persantine-Aspirin Trial in cerebral ischemia. Part II: endpoint result. Stroke 1985; 16:406–415.
68. NASCET Investigators. Benefit of carotid endarterectomy for patients with high-grade stenosis of the internal carotid artery. NINDS Clinical Alert 1991.
69. North American Symptomatic Carotid Endarterectomy Trial Collaborators. Beneficial effect of carotid endarterectomy in symptomatic patients with high grade stenosis. N Engl J Med 1991; 325:445–453.
70. Barnett H, et al. Benefit of carotid endarterectomy in patients with symptomatic moderate or severe stenosis. N Engl J Med 1998; 339(20):1415–1425.
71. MRC European Carotid Surgery Trial. Interim results for symptomatic patients with severe (70–99%) or with mild (0-29%) carotid stenosis. Lancet 1991; 337:1235–1243.
72. European Carotid Surgery Trialists Collaborative Group. Randomised trial of endarterectomy for recently symptomatic carotid stenosis: final results of the MRC European Carotid Surgery Trial (ECST). Lancet 1998; 351:1379–1387.
73. Rothwell P, Gutnikov S, Warlow C. Reanalysis of the final results of the European Carotid Surgery Trial. Stroke 2003; 34:514–532.
74. Mayberg MR, et al. Carotid endarterectomy and prevention of cerebral ischemia in symptomatic carotid stenosis. J Am Med Assoc 1991; 266:3289–3294.
75. Wylie E, Hein M, Adams J. Intracranial hemorrhage following surgical revascularization for treatment of acute strokes. J Neurosurg 1964; 21:212–215.
76. Hunter J, et al. Emergency operation for acute cerebral ischemia due to carotid artery obstruction; review of 26 cases. Ann Surg 1965; 162:901–905.
77. Millikan CH, McDowell FH. Treatment of progressing stroke. Prog Cardiovasc Dis 1980; 22:397–414.

78. Najafi H, et al. Emergency carotid thromboendarterectomy, surgical indications and results. Arch Surg 1971; 103:610–613.
79. Goldstone J, Moore WS. A new look at emergency carotid artery operations for the treatment of cerebrovascular insufficiency. Stroke 1978; 9:599–602.
80. Mentzer R, et al. Emergency carotid endarterectomy for fluctuating neurological deficits. Surgery 1981; 89:60–66.
81. Walters BB, Ojemann RG, Heros RC. Emergency carotid endarterectomy. J Neurosurg 1987; 66:817–823.
82. Meyer FB, et al. Emergency carotid endarterectomy for patients with acute carotid occlusion and profound neurological deficits. Ann Surg 1986:82–89.
83. Tretter JF, et al. Perioperative risk and late outcome of nonelective carotid endarterectomy. J Vasc Surg 1999; 30(4): 618–631.
84. McPherson CM, et al. Early carotid endarterectomy for critical carotid artery stenosis after thrombolysis therapy in acute ischemic stroke in the middle cerebral artery. Stroke 2001; 32:2075.
85. Eckstein H–H, et al. Carotid endarterectomy and intracranial thrombolysis: simultaneous and staged procedures in ischemic stroke. J Vasc Surg 1999; 29(3): 459–471.
86. Hugenholtz H, Elgie R. Carotid thromboendarterectomy: a reappraisal. J Neurosurg 1980; 53:776–783.
87. Hafner C, Tew JM. Surgical management of the totally occluded internal carotid artery: a ten-year study. Surgery 1981; 89:710–717.
88. Thompson JE, Austin D, Patman R. Endarterectomy of the totally occluded carotid artery for stroke. Arch Surg 1967; 95:791–801.
89. Shucart WA, Garrido E. Reopening some occluded carotid arteries. Report of four cases. J Neurosurg 1976; 45:442–446.
90. Kusonaki T, Rowed D, Tator C. Thromboendarterectomy for total occlusion of the internal carotid artery: a reappraisal of risks, success rate, and potential benefits. Stroke 1978; 9:34–38.
91. McCormick PW, et al. Thromboendarterectomy of the symptomatic occluded internal carotid artery. J Neurosurg 1992; 76:752–758.
92. Kasper GC, et al. Carotid thromboendarterectomy for recent total occlusion of the internal carotid artery. J Vasc Surg 2001; 33(2): 242–250.
93. Paty PSK, et al. Surgical treatment of internal carotid artery occlusion. J Vasc Surg 2003; 37(4): 785–788.
94. Barnett HJM, Peerless SJ, Kaufmann JCE. "Stump" of internal carotid artery—a source for further embolic cerebral ischemia. Stroke 1978; 9:448–456.
95. Countee RW, Vijoyanathan T. Intracranial embolization via external carotid artery: report of a case with angiographic documentation. Stroke 1980; 11:465–468.
96. Watts C. External carotid artery embolus from the internal carotid artery "stump" during angiography: case report. Stroke 1982; 13:515–517.
97. Honeycutt JH, Loftus CM. Carotid stump syndromes and external revascularization. In: Loftus C, Kresowik T, eds. Carotid Artery Surgery. New York: Thieme Medical Publishers, 2000.
98. Rosenthal D, Stanton P, Lamis P. Carotid endarterectomy: the unreliability of intraoperative monitoring in patients having had a stroke or reversible ischemic neurological deficit. Arch Surg 1981; 116:1569–1575.
99. Moore W, Yee J, Hall A. Collateral cerebral blood pressure: an index to tolerance to temporary carotid occlusion. Arch Surg 1973; 106:520–523.
100. Little JR, Moufarrij N, Furlan AJ. Early carotid endarterectomy after cerebral infarction. Neurosurgery 1989; 24:334–338.
101. Piotrowski J, et al. Timing of carotid endarterectomy after acute stroke. J Vasc Surg 1990; 11:45–52.
102. Pritz MB. Carotid endarterectomy after recent stroke: preliminary observations in patients undergoing early operation. Neurosurgery 1986; 19:604–609.
103. Anson J, Heiserman J, Drayer B. Surgical decisions on the basis of magnetic resonance angiography of the carotid arteries. Neurosurgery 1993; 32:335–343.
104. LeClerc X, et al. Computed tomography angiography for the evaluation of carotid artery stenosis. Stroke 1995; 26:1577–1581.
105. Qureshi AI, et al. Role of conventional angiography in evaluation of patients with carotid artery stenosis demonstrated by Doppler ultrasound in general practice. Stroke 2001; 32:2287.

106. Gomez C. Carotid plaque morphology and risk for stroke. Stroke 1990; 21:148–151.
107. Wechsler L. Ulceration and carotid artery disease. Stroke 1988; 19:650–653.
108. Eliasziw M, Striefler J, Fox A. Significance of plague ulceration in patients with high-grade carotid stenosis. Stroke 1994; 25:304–308.
109. Lennihan L, Kupsky W, Mohr J. Lack of association between carotid plague hematoma and ischemic cerebral symptoms. Stroke 1987; 18:879–881.
110. Biller J, et al. Intraluminal clot of the carotid artery. Surg Neurol 1986; 25:467–477.
111. Heros RC. Carotid endarterectomy in patients with intraluminal thrombus. Stroke 1990; 19:667–668.
112. Loftus C. Propagating intraluminal carotid thrombus—surgery or anticoagulation? In: Loftus C, Kresowik T, eds. Carotid Artery Surgery. New York: Thieme Medical Publishers, 2000:321–328.
113. Buchan A, et al. Intraluminal thrombus in the cerebral circulation: implications for surgical management. Stroke 1988, 19:681–698.
114. Fields W, Lemak N. Joint study of extracranial arterial occlusion. X. Internal carotid artery occlusion. J Am Med Assoc 1976; 235:2734–2738.
115. Callow A, et al. Protection of the high risk carotid endarterectomy patient by continuous electroencephalography. J Cardiovasc Surg 1978; 19:55–64.
116. Whittemore A, et al. Routine electroencephalographic (EEG) monitoring during carotid endarterectomy. Ann Surg 1982; 197:707–713.
117. Baker W, Dorner D, Barnes R. Carotid endarterectomy: is an indwelling shunt necessary? Surgery 1977; 82:321–326.
118. Littooy F, Halstuk K, Mamdani M. Factors influencing morbidity of carotid endarterectomy without a shunt. Am Surg 1984; 50:350–353.
119. Andersen C, Rich N, Collins G. Unilateral internal carotid artery occlusion: special considerations. Stroke 1977; 8:669–671.
120. Patterson RH. Technique of Carotid Endarterectomy. In: Smith RR, ed. Stroke and the Extracranial Vessels. New York: Raven Press, 1984:177–185.
121. Sachs S, Fullenwider T, Smith R. Does contralateral carotid occlusion influence neurologic fate of carotid endarterectomy? Surgery 1984; 96:839–844.
122. Redekop G, Ferguson G. Correlation of contralateral stenosis and intraoperative electroencephalogram change with risk of stroke during carotid endarterectomy. Neurosurgery 1992; 30:191–194.
123. Loftus CM., Overview of shunt controversy. In: Loftus C, Kresowik T, eds. Carotid Artery Surgery. New York: Thieme Medical Publishers, 2000.
124. Barnett H. Status report on the North American Symptomatic Carotid Surgery Trial. J Mal Vasc 1993; 18:202–208.
125. Rutgers DR, et al. Sustained bilateral hemodynamic benefit of contralateral carotid endarterectomy in patients with symptomatic internal carotid artery occlusion. Stroke 2001; 32:728.
126. Roederer G, Langlois Y, Chan A. Is siphon disease important in predicting outcome of carotid endarterectomy? Arch Surg 1983; 118:1177–1181.
127. Schuler J, Flanigan D, Lim L. The effect of carotid siphon stenosis on stroke rate, death, and relief of symptoms following elective carotid endarterectomy. Surgery 1982; 92:1058–1067.
128. Day A, Rhoton A, Quisling R. Resolving siphon stenosis following endarterectomy. Stroke 1980; 11:278–281.
129. Little J, Sawhny B, Weinstein M. Pseudo-tandem stenosis of the internal carotid artery. Neurosurgery 1980; 7:574–577.
130. Kappelle LJ, et al. Importance of intracranial atherosclerotic disease in patients with symptomatic stenosis of the internal carotid artery. Stroke 1999; 30:282–286.
131. Adams H. Carotid stenosis and coexisting ipsilateral intracranial aneurysm. Arch Neurol 1977; 34:515–516.
132. Ladowski J, Webster M, Yonas H. Carotid endarterectomy in patients with asymptomatic intracranial aneurysms. Ann Surg 1984; 200:70–73.
133. Stern J, Whelan M, Brisman R. Management of extracranial carotid stenosis and intracranial aneurysms. J Neurosurg 1979; 51:147–150.
134. Julien T, Hodge C. Simultaneous carotid occlusive disease and intracranial aneurysm. In: Loftus C, Kresowik T, eds. Carotid Artery Surgery. New York: Thieme Medical Publishers, 2000:131–137.

135. Salvian A, Baker J, Machleder H. Cause and noninvasive detection of restenosis after endarterectomy. Am J Surg 1983; 146:29–34.
136. Piepgras D, Sundt T, Marsh W. Recurrent carotid stenosis: results and complications of 57 operations. In: Sundt T, ed. Occlusive Cerebrovascular Disease: Diagnosis and Surgical Management. Philadelphia: WB Saunders, 1987:286–297.
137. Clagett GP, et al. Etiologic factors for recurrent carotid artery stenosis. Surgery 1983; 2:313–318.
138. Dempsey RJ, Moore R, Cordero S. Factors leading to early reoccurrence of carotid plaque after carotid endarterectomy. Surg Neurol 1995; 43:278–283.
139. AbuRahma AF, et al. Redo carotid endarterectomy versus primary carotid endarterectomy. Stroke 2001; 32(12): 2787.
140. O'Hara PJ, et al. Reoperation for recurrent carotid stenosis: early results and late outcome in 199 patients. J Vasc Surg 2001; 34(1): 5–12.
141. Yadav JS, et al. Protected carotid-artery stenting versus endarterectomy in high-risk patients. N Engl J Med 2004; 351:1493–1501.
142. Graor R, Hertzer N. Management of coexistent carotid artery and coronary artery disease. In Current Concepts of Cerebrovascular Disease and Stroke. 1988; 19–23.
143. Jones R, et al. Concomitant carotid and coronary disease. Patient Care 1992; 15:49–66.
144. Brown KR, et al. Multistate population-based outcomes of combined carotid endarterectomy and coronary artery bypass. J Vasc Surg 2003; 37(1): 32–39.
145. Cosgrove D, Hertzer N, Loop F. Surgical management of synchronous carotid and coronary artery disease. J Vasc Surg 1986; 3:690–692.
146. Newman, D, Hicks R. Combined carotid and coronary artery surgery: a review of the literature. Ann Thorac Surg 1988; 45:574–581.
147. Loftus CM, Kresowik TF. Anatomical basis and technique of carotid endarterectomy. In: Loftus C, Kresowik T, eds. Carotid Artery Surgery. New York: Thieme Medical Publishers, 2000.
148. Rich, N, Hobson R. Carotid endarterectomy under regional anesthesia. Am Surg 1975; 41:253–259.
149. Craen R, et al. Anesthesia for carotid endarterectomy, the North American practice at 50 centres: NASCET study results. Anesth Analg 1993; 76:S61.
150. Cheng M, Theard M, Tempelhoff R. Anesthesia for carotid endarterectomy: a survey. J Neurosurg Anesth 1997; 9:211–216.
151. Loftus C. Carotid endarterectomy. In: Loftus C, Batjer H, eds. Techniques in Neurosurgery. Philadelphia: Lippincott, Williams and Wilkins, 1997.
152. Loftus C. Technical aspects of carotid endarterectomy with Hemashield patch graft. Neurologia medico-chirurgia (Tokyo) 1997; 37:805–818.
153. Loftus C. Anesthesia for carotid endarterectomy: general vs. local? In: Bederson J, Tuhrim S, eds. Treatment of Carotid Disease: A Practitioner's Manual. Park Ridge, IL: AANS, 1998:181–190.
154. Loftus C. Surgical anatomy, technique, and indications for carotid endarterectomy. In: Matsuno H, ed. Proceedings of the 12th Microsurgical Anatomy Seminar Program. Tokyo: SciMed Publications, 1998.
155. Loftus C, Surgical management of extracranial carotid artery disease. Surgery for Cerebral Stroke (Japan) 1999; 27:7–13.
156. Loftus C. Surgical management of extracranial carotid stenosis. In Schmidek H, Sweet W, eds. Operative Neurosurgical Techniques. Philadelphia: WB Saunders, 2000:1067–1079.
157. Loftus CM. High-risk carotid endarterectomy and high-risk carotid surgery: is surgery or stenting the best choice. In Watanabe K (ed)., Developments in Neuroscience, Proceedings of the 2nd Mt. Bandai Symposium for Neuroscience 2001. International Congress Series 2002; 1247:319–326.
158. Loftus C, Biller J. Acute cerebral ischemia. Surgical management. Contemp Neurosurg 1994; 16:26.
159. Loftus C, Biller J. Acute medical and surgical management of stroke, in Tindall G, Cooper P, Barrow D, eds. The Practice of Neurosurgery. Baltimore: Williams and Wilkins, 1995.
160. Loftus C, Robertson S. Technique of carotid endarterectomy with special emphasis on Hemashield patch graft technique. In: Monduzzi ed. Proceedings of the 11th International Congress of Neurological Surgery. Bologna, IT, 1997: 1871–1875.
161. Loftus C, Stanfield M. Carotid endarterectomy. in Batjer H, Loftus C, eds. Textbook of Neurological Surgery. Philadelphia: Lippincott, Williams and Wilkins, 2003.

162. Loftus CM. Technique of carotid endarterectomy. Contemp Neurosurg 1988; 10(5): 1–6.

163. Loftus CM. Monitoring during extracranial carotid reconstruction. In: Loftus CM, Traynelis VC, eds. Intraoperative monitoring techniques in neurosurgery. New York: McGraw-Hill, 1994:3–8.

164. Loftus CM. Carotid endarterectomy: conventional and microsurgical techniques. Congress of Neurological Surgeons, Video Perspectives in Neurological Surgery Series. St. Louis, Missouri: Quality Medical Publishing, 1996.

165. Loftus CM. Carotid endarterectomy: how the operation is done. Clin Neurosurg 1997; 44:243–265.

166. Loftus CM. Technical fundamentals, monitoring, and shunt use during carotid endarterectomy. Techn Neurosurg 1997; 3:16–24.

167. Loftus CM, Quest DO. Technical controversies in carotid artery surgery. Neurosurgery 1987; 20:490–495.

168. Loftus CM, Quest DO. Technical issues in carotid surgery 1995. Neurosurgery 1995; 36:629–647.

169. Collier P, et al. Carotid endarterectomy clinical pathway: an innovative approach. Am J Med Qual 1995; 10:38–47.

170. Harbaugh KS, Harbaugh RE. Early discharge after carotid endarterectomy. Neurosurgery 1995; 37:219–225.

171. Allen B, et al. The influence of anesthetic technqiue on perioperative complications after carotid endarterectomy. J Vasc Surg 1994; 19:833–843.

172. Sternbach Y, et al. Hemodynamic benefits of regional anesthesia for carotid endarterectomy. J Vasc Surg 2002; 35:333–339.

173. Sbarigia E, et al. Locoregional versus general anesthesia in carotid surgery: is there an impact on perioperative myocardial ischemia? Results of a prospective monocentric randomized trial. J Vasc Surg 1999; 30(1): 131–138.

174. Corson J, et al. The influence of anesthetic choice on carotid endarterectomy outcome. Arch Surg 1987; 122:807–812.

175. Forssell C, et al. Local versus general anesthesia in carotid surgery. A prospective randomized study. Eur J Vasc Surg 1989; 3:503–509.

176. Wellman B, et al. The differences in electroencephalographic changes in local versus general anesthesia carotid endarterectomy patients. Neurosurgery 1998; 43:769–775.

177. Wellman BJ, et al. The differences in electroencephalographic changes in awake versus anesthetized carotid endarterectomy patients. J Neurosurg 1997; 86:405A.

178. Shah D, et al. Carotid endarterectomy in awake patients: Its safety, acceptability and outcome. J Vasc Surg 1994; 19:1015–1020.

179. Palmer M. Comparison of regional and general anesthesia for carotid endarterectomy. Am J Surg 1989; 157:329–330.

180. Harbaugh RE. Carotid surgery under local anesthesia. Techniques in Neurosurgery 1997; 3:25–33.

181. Benjamin M, et al. Awake patient monitoring to determine the need for shunting during carotid endarterectomy. Surgery 1993; 114:673–681.

182. Spielberger L, et al. Hand-held toy squeaker during carotid endarterectomy in the awake patient. Arch Surg 1979; 114:103–104.

183. Steed D, Peitzman A, Grundy B. Causes of stroke in carotid endarterectomy. Surgery 1982; 92:634–641.

184. Whittemore A, Carotid endarterectomy. An alternative approach. Arch Surg 1980; 115:940–942.

185. Erwin D, Pick M, Taylor G. Anaesthesia for carotid artery surgery. Anaesthesia 1980; 35:246–249.

186. Connolly J, Kwaan J, Stemmer E. Improved results with carotid endarterectomy. Ann Surg 1977; 186:334–342.

187. Tiberio G, Guilini S, Floriani M. Intra-operative control of carotid thromboendarterectomy by Doppler spectrum analysis. J Cardiovasc Surg 1984; 25:361–364.

188. Michenfelder J. Anesthetic and pharmacologic management. In: Meyer F, ed. Sundt's Occlusive Cerebrovascular Disease. 2nd ed. Philadelphia: W.B. Saunders, 1994:171–178.

189. Hafner C, Evans W. Carotid endarterectomy with local anesthesia: results and advantages. J Vasc Surg 1988; 7:232–239.

190. Davies M, et al. Carotid endarterectomy under cervical plexus block—a prospective clinical audit. Anaesth Intens Care 1990; 18:219–223.

191. Gelb A. Anesthetic considerations for carotid endarterectomy. Int Anesth Clin 1984; 22:153–164.
192. Wells B, Keats A, Cooley D. Increased tolerance to cerebral ischemia produced by general anesthesia during temporary carotid occlusion. Surgery 1963; 54:216–223.
193. Fourcade H, et al. The effects of CO_2 and systemic hypertension on cerebral perfusion pressure during carotid endarterectomy. Anesthesiology 1970; 33:383–390.
194. Pistolese G, et al. Effects of hypercapnia on cerebral blood flow during the clamping of the carotid arteries in surgical management of cerebrovascular insufficiency. Neurology 1971; 21:95–100.
195. Boysen G, et al. The effect of $PaCO_2$ on regional cerebral blood flow and internal carotid arterial pressure during carotid clamping. Anesthesiology 1971; 35:286–300.
196. Lassen N, Palvolgyi R. Cerebral steal during hypercapnia and the inverse reaction during hypocapnia observed by the 113 xenon technique in man. Scan J Clin Lab Invest 1968. XIII:(Suppl. 102):D.
197. Muhonen M, et al. Mechanism of redistribution of cerebral blood flow during hypercarbia and seizures. Am J Physiol (Heart Circ Physiol) 1994; 35:H2074–2081.
198. Muhonen M, et al. Mechanism of cerebral vascular "steal" phenomenon during hypercarbia and seizures. Stroke 1992; 23:139.
199. Baker W, et al. An evaluation of hypocarbia and hypercarbia during carotid endarterectomy. Stroke 1976; 7:451–454.
200. Smith A, Wollman H. Cerebral blood flow and metabolism: effects of anesthetic drugs and techniques. Anesthesiology 1972; 36:378–400.
201. Moore W, Hall A. Carotid artery back pressure: a test of cerebral tolerance to temporary clip occlusion. Arch Surg 1969; 99:702–710.
202. Hunter G, et al. The accuracy of carotid back pressure as an index for shunt requirements: a reappraisal. Stroke 1982; 13:319–326.
203. Hays R, Levinson S, Wylie E. Intraoperative measurement of carotid back pressure as a guide to operative management for carotid endarterectomy. Surgery 1972; 72:953–960.
204. Hobson R, et al. Carotid artery back pressure and endarterectomy under regional anesthesia. Arch Surg 1974; 109:682–687.
205. Archie J, Hemodynamics of carotid back pressure and cerebral flow during endarterectomy. J Surg Res 1977; 23:223–232.
206. Archie J, Feldtman R. Determinants of cerebral perfusion pressure during carotid endarterectomy. Arch Surg 1982; 117:319–322.
207. Kwaan H, Peterson G, Connolly J. Stump pressure: an unreliable guide for shunting during carotid endarterectomy. Arch Surg 1980; 115:1083–1085.
208. Sublett J, Seidenberg A, Hobson R. Internal carotid artery stump pressures during regional anesthesia. Anesthesiology 1974; 41:505–508.
209. Beebe H, Pearson J, Coatsworth J. Comparison of carotid artery stump pressure and EEG monitoring in carotid endarterectomy. Am Surg 1978; 44:655–660.
210. Boysen G. Cerebral blood flow measurement as a safeguard during carotid endarterectomy. Stroke 1971; 2:1–10.
211. Kelly J, et al. Failure of carotid stump pressure: its incidence as a predictor for a temporary shunt during carotid endarterectomy. Arch Surg 1979; 114:1361–1366.
212. McKay R, et al. Internal carotid artery stump pressure and cerebral blood flow during carotid endarterectomy: modification by halothane, enflurane, and innovar. Anesthesiology 1976; 45:390–399.
213. Rowed D, Vilaghy M. Intraoperative regional cerebral blood flow during carotid endarterectomy. Can J Neurol Sci 1981; 8:235–241.
214. Messick J, Sharbrough F, Sundt TM. Selective shunting on the basis of EEG and regional CBF monitoring during carotid endarterectomy. Int Anesth Clin 1984; 22:137–145.
215. Sundt T, et al. Correlation of cerebral blood flow and electroencephalographic changes during carotid endarterectomy: with results of surgery and hemodynamics of cerebral ischemia. Mayo Clin Proc 1981; 56:533–543.
216. Sundt T. The ischemic tolerance of neural tissue and the need for monitoring and selective shunting during carotid endarterectomy. Stroke 1983; 14:93–98.
217. Trojaborg W, Boysen G. Relationship between EEG, regional cerebral blood flow and internal carotid artery pressure during carotid endarterectomy. Electroenceph Clin Neurophysiol 1973; 34:61–69.

218. Morawetz R, et al. Correlation of cerebral blood flow and EEG during carotid occlusion for endarterectomy (without shunting) and neurologic outcome. Surgery 1984; 96:184–189.

219. Benichou H, et al. Pre- and intraoperative transcranial Doppler: prediction and surveillance of tolerance to carotid clamping. Ann Vasc Surg 1991; 5:21–25.

220. Schneider P, Rossman M, Torem S. Transcranial Doppler in the management of extracranial cerebrovascular disease: implications and diagnosis and monitoring. J Vasc Surg 1988; 7:223–231.

221. Bergeron P, et al. Stroke prevention during carotid surgery in high risk patients (value of transcranial Doppler and local anesthesia). J Cardiovasc Surg 1991; 32:713–719.

222. Jorgensen L, Schroeder T. Transcranial Doppler for detection of cerebral ischaemia during carotid endarterectomy. Eur J Vasc Surg 1992; 6:142–147.

223. Naylor A, et al. Transcranial Doppler monitoring during carotid endarterectomy. Br J Surg 1991; 78:1264–1268.

224. Padayachee T, et al. Transcranial Doppler assessment of cerebral collateral during carotid endarterectomy. Br J Surg 1987; 74:260–262.

225. Spencer M, Thomas G, Moehring M. Relation between middle cerebral artery blood flow velocity and stump pressure during carotid endarterectomy. Stroke 1992; 23:439–445.

226. Halsey J, McDowell H, Selman S. Transcranial Doppler and rCBF compared in carotid endarterectomy. Stroke 1986; 17:1206–1208.

227. Thiel A, et al. Transcranial Doppler sonography and somatosensory evoked potential monitoring in carotid surgery. Eur J Vasc Surg 1990; 4:597–602.

228. Halsey JH. Risks and benefits of shunting in carotid endarterectomy. Stroke 1992:1583–1587.

229. Prioleau W, Aiken A, Hairston P. Carotid endarterectomy: neurologic complications as related to surgical techniques. Ann Surg 1977; 185:678–683.

230. Jansen C, et al. Carotid endarterectomy with transcranial Doppler and electroencephalographic monitoring: a prospective study in 130 operations. Stroke 1993; 24:665–669.

231. Marcus H. Transcranial Doppler detection of circulating cerebral emboli. A review. Stroke 1993; 24:1246–1250.

232. Georgiadis D, Grosset D, Lees K. Transhemispheric passage of microemboli in patients with unilateral internal carotid artery occlusion. Stroke 1993; 24:1664–1666.

233. Spencer M, et al. Detection of middle cerebral artery emboli during carotid endarterectomy using transcranial Doppler ultrasonography. Stroke 1990; 21:414–423.

234. Jansen C, et al. Impact of microembolism and hemodynamic changes in the brain during carotid endarterectomy. Stroke 1994; 25:992–997.

235. Padayachee T, et al. Monitoring cerebral perfusion during carotid endarterectomy. J Cardiovasc Surg 1990; 31:112–114.

236. Laman D, et al. Intraoperative internal carotid artery restenosis detected by transcranial Doppler monitoring. Br J Surg 1989; 76:1315–1316.

237. Powers A, Smith R. Hyperperfusion syndrome after carotid endarterectomy: a transcranial Doppler evaluation. Neurosurgery 1990; 26:56–60.

238. Ackerstaff R, et al. The significance of microemboli detection by means of transcranial Doppler monitoring in carotid endarterectomy. J Vasc Surg 1996; 23(4): 734–736.

239. Spencer MP. Transcranial Doppler monitoring and causes of stroke from carotid endarterectomy. Stroke 1997; 28:685–691.

240. Gee W, McDonald K, Kaupp H. Carotid endarterectomy shunting: effectiveness determined by operative ocular pneumoplethysmography. Arch Surg 1979; 114:720–721.

241. Pearce H, et al. Continuous oculoplethysmographic monitoring during carotid endarterectomy. Am J Surg 1979; 138:733–735.

242. Pearce H, Becchetti J, Brown H. Supraorbital photoplethysmographic monitoring during carotid endarterectomy with the use of an internal shunt: an added dimension of safety. Surgery 1980; 87:339–342.

243. Blaisdell F, Routine operative arteriography following carotid endarterectomy. Surgery 1978; 83:114–115.

244. Blaisdell F, Lim R, Hall A. Technical result of carotid endarterectomy: arteriographic assessment. Am J Surg 1967; 114:239–246.

245. Plecha F, Pories W. Intraoperative angiography in the immediate assessment of arterial reconstruction. Arch Surg 1972; 105:902–907.

246. Rosental J, Gaspar M, Movius H. Intraoperative arteriography in carotid thromboendarterectomy. Arch Surg 1973; 106:806–808.

247. Scott S, Sethi G, Bridgman A. Perioperative stroke during carotid endarterectomy: the value of intraoperative angiography. J Cardiovasc Surg 1982; 23:353–358.

248. Jernigan W, Fulton R, Hammon J. The efficacy of routine completion operative angiography in reducing the incidence of perioperative stroke associated with carotid endarterectomy. Surgery 1984; 96:831–838.

249. Andersen C, Collins G, Rich N. Routine operative arteriography during carotid endarterectomy: a reassessment. Surgery 1978; 83:67–73.

250. Wassmann H, Fischdick G, Jain K. Cerebral protection during carotid endarterectomy-EEG monitoring as a guide to the use of intraluminal shunts. Acta Neurochirurgica 1984; 71:99–108.

251. Zierler R, Bandyk D, Berni G. Intraoperative pulsed Doppler assessment of carotid endarterectomy. J Ultrasound Med Biol 1983; 9:65–71.

252. Seifert K, Blackshear W. Continuous-wave Doppler in the intraoperative assessment of carotid endarterectomy. J Vasc Surg 1985; 2:817–820.

253. Perez-Borja C, Meyer J. Electroencephalographic monitoring during reconstructive surgery of the neck vessels. Electroenceph Clin Neurophysiol 1965; 18:162–169.

254. Harris E, et al. Continuous electroencephalographic monitoring during carotid endarterectomy. Surgery 1967; 62:441–447.

255. Baker J, et al. An evaluation of electroencephalographic monitoring for carotid study. Surgery 1975; 78:787–794.

256. Marshall B, Lougheed W. The use of electroencephalographic monitoring during carotid endarterectomy, as an indicator for the application of a temporary bypass. Can Anaes Soc J 1969; 16:331–335.

257. Horton D, et al. The virtues of continuous EEG monitoring during carotid endarterectomy. Aust N Z Med 1974; 4:32–40.

258. Green R. Angiographic and clinical correlates of shunt requirements during carotid endarterectomy. Stroke 1982; 13:120.

259. String T, Callahan A. The critical manipulable variables of hemispheric low flow during carotid surgery. Surgery 1983; 93:46–49.

260. Markand ON. Continuous assessment of cerebral function with EEG and somatosensory evoked potential techniques during extracranial vascular reconstruction. In: Loftus C, Traynelis V, eds. Intraoperative Monitoring Techniques in Neurosurgery. Philadelphia: McGraw-Hill, 1994.

261. Chiappa K, et al. The usefulness of EEG monitoring during carotid endarterectomy. Neurology 1978; 28:341.

262. Blume W, Ferguson G, McNeill D. Significance of EEG changes at carotid endarterectomy. Stroke 1986; 17:891–897.

263. Chiappa K, Young R. Carotid endarterectomy monitoring with a dedicated minicomputer. Electroenceph Clin Neurophys 1977; 43:518.

264. Chiappa K, Burke S, Young R. Results of electroencephalographic monitoring during 367 carotid endarterectomies: use of a dedicated minicomputer. Stroke 1979; 10:381–388.

265. Myers R, Stockard J, Saidman L. Monitoring of cerebral perfusion during anesthesia by time-compressed Fourier analysis of the electroencephalogram. Stroke 1977; 8:331–337.

266. Rampil I, et al. Prognostic value of computerized EEG analysis during carotid endarterectomy. Anesth Analg 1983; 62:186–192.

267. Rampil I, et al. Computerized electroencephalogram monitoring and carotid artery shunting. Neurosurgery 1983; 13:276–279.

268. Amantini A, et al. Selective shunting based on somatosensory evoked potential monitoring during carotid endarterectomy. Inter Angio 1987; 6:387–390.

269. Amantini A, et al. Monitoring of somatosensory evoked potentials during carotid endarterectomy. J Neurol 1992; 239:241–247.

270. DeVleeschauwer P, Horsch S, Matamoros R. Monitoring of somatosensory evoked potentials in carotid surgery: results, usefulness, and limitations of the method. Ann Vasc Surg 1988; 2:63–68.

271. Haupt W, Horsch S. Evoked potential monitoring in carotid surgery: a review of 994 cases. Neurology 1992; 42:835–838.

272. Horsch S, DeVleeschauwer P, Ktenidis K. Intraoperative assessment of cerebral ischemia during carotid surgery. J Neurol 1991; 239:241–247.

273. Jacobs L, et al. Long-latency somatosensory evoked potentials during carotid endarterectomy. Am Surg 1983; 49:338–344.

274. Kearse L, Brown E, McPeck K. Somatosensory evoked potentials sensitivity to electroencephalography for cerebral ischemia during carotid endarterectomy. Stroke 1992; 23:498–505.

275. Lam A, et al. Monitoring electrophysiologic function during carotid endarterectomy: a comparison of somatosensory evoked potentials and conventional electroencephalogram. Anesthesiology 1991; 75:15–21.

276. Tiberio G, et al. Monitoring of somatosensory evoked potentials during carotid endarterectomy: relationship with different haemodynamic parameters and clinical outcome. Eur J Vasc Surg 1991; 5:647–653.

277. Russ W, et al. Intraoperative somatosensory evoked potentials as a prognostic factor of neurologic state after carotid endarterectomy. Thorac Cardiovasc Surg 1985; 33:392–396.

278. Markand ON, et al. Monitoring of somatosensory evoked responses during carotid endarterectomy. Arch Neurol 1984; 41:375–378.

279. Schweiger H, Kamp HD, Dinkel M. Somatosensory-evoked potentials during carotid artery surgery: experience in 400 operations. Surgery 1991; 109:602–609.

280. Gautier P, et al. Changes in somatosensory evoked responses during carotid endarterectomy related to head position. Anesth Analg 1991; 73:649–652.

281. Kirkpatrick PJ, et al. An observational study of near-infrared spectroscopy during carotid endarterectomy. J Neurosurg 1995; 82:756–763.

282. Kuroda S, et al. Near-infrared monitoring of cerebral oxygenation state during carotid endarterectomy. Surg Neurol 1996; 45:450–458.

283. Kirkpatrick P, Minhas P. Near-infrared spectroscopy during carotid surgery. in Loftus C, Kresowik T, eds. Carotid Artery Surgery. New York: Thieme, 2000:447–456.

284. Smielewski P, et al. Clinical evaluation of near-infrared spectroscopy for testing cerebrovascular reactivity in patients with carotid artery disease. Stroke 1997; 28:331–338.

285. Loftus C. Design characteristics and clinical application of a newly designed carotid artery shunt. Neurological Research 2000; 22:443–448.

286. Aufiero TX, et al. Hemodynamic performance of carotid artery shunts. Am J Surg 1989; 158:95–100.

287. Benoit B, Navavi N. The "routine" use of intraluminal shunting in carotid endarterectomy. Can J Neurol Sci 1978; 5:339.

288. Giannotta SL, Dicks RE, Kindt GW. Carotid endarterectomy: technical improvements. Neurosurgery 1980; 7:309–312.

289. Javid H, et al. Seventeen year experience with routine shunting in carotid artery surgery. World J Surg 1979; 3:167–177.

290. Schiro J, et al. Routine use of a shunt for carotid endarterectomy. Am J Surg 1981; 142:735–738.

291. Thompson J. Protection of the brain during carotid endarterectomy. Int Anesth Clin 1984; 22:123–128.

292. Lindsey R. A simple solution for determining shunt flow during carotid endarterectomy. Anesthesiology 1984; 61:215–216.

293. Loftus CM, et al. Cervical carotid dissection following carotid endarterectomy: a complication of indwelling shunt? Neurosurgery 1986; 19:441–445.

294. Gross CE, et al. Use of anticoagulants, electroencephalographic monitoring, and barbiturate cerebral protection in carotid endarterectomy. Neurosurgery 1981; 9:1–5.

295. Spetzler RF, et al. Microsurgical endarterectomy under barbiturate protection: a prospective study. J Neurosurg 1986; 51:147–150.

296. Allen G, Preziosi T. Carotid endarterectomy: a prospective study of its efficacy and safety. Medicine 1980; 60:298–309.

297. Bland J, Lazar M. Carotid endarterectomy without shunt. Neurosurgery 1981; 8:153–157.

298. Ferguson GG. Intra-operative monitoring and internal shunts: are they necessary in carotid endarterectomy? Stroke 1982; 13:287–289.

299. Ferguson GG. Carotid endarterectomy: indications and surgical technique. Int Anesth Clin 1984; 22:113–121.

300. Ferguson GG. Shunt almost never. Int Anesth Clin 1984; 22:147–152.

301. Ferguson GG. Carotid endarterectomy. To shunt or not to shunt? Arch Neurol 1986; 43:615–617.

302. Ott D, et al. Carotid endarterectomy without temporary intraluminal shunt. Ann Surg 1980; 191:708–714.

303. Whitney D, et al. Carotid artery surgery without a temporary indwelling shunt. Arch Surg 1980; 115:1393–1399.

304. Ojemann RG, Heros RC. Carotid endarterectomy. To shunt or not to shunt? Arch Neurol 1986; 43:617–618.

305. Rosenthal D, et al. Carotid endarterectomy after reversible ischemic neurologic deficit or stroke: is it of value? J Vasc Surg 1988; 8:527–534.

306. Green R, et al. Benefits, shortcomings, and costs of EEG monitoring. Ann Surg 1985; 201:785–792.

307. Hayes P, et al. The Pruitt-Inahara shunt maintains mean middle cerebral artery velocities within 10% of preoperative values during carotid endarterectomy. J Vasc Surg 2000; 32(2): 299–306.

308. Little J, Bryerton B, Furlan A. Saphenous vein patch grafts in carotid endarterectomy. J Neurosurg 1984; 61:743–747.

309. Archie JP. Reoperations for carotid artery stenosis: role of primary and secondary reconstructions. J Vasc Surg 2001; 33(3): 495–503.

310. Kresowik T, et al. Multistate utilization, processes, and outcomes of carotid endarterectomy. J Vasc Surg 2001; 33(2): 227–235.

311. AbuRahma AF, et al. Prospective randomized trial of bilateral carotid endarterectomies. Stroke 1999; 30:1185–1189.

312. Archie JP. Carotid endarterectomy outcome with vein or Dacron graft patch angioplasty and internal carotid artery shortening. J Vasc Surg 1999; 29(4): 654–664.

313. Yamamoto Y, et al. Complications resulting from saphenous vein patch graft after carotid endarterectomy. Neurosurgery 1996; 39:670–676.

314. Hayes PD, et al. Randomized trial of vein versus Dacron patching during carotid endarterectomy: influence of patch type on postoperative embolization. J Vasc Surg 2001; 33(5): 994–1000.

315. O'Hara P, et al. A prospective randomized study of saphenous vein patching versus synthetic patching during carotid endarterectomy. J Vasc Surg 2002; 35(2): 324–332.

316. AbuRahma AF, et al. Prospective randomized study of carotid endarterectomy with polytetrafluorethylene versus collagen-impregnated Dacron (Hemashield) patching; Perioperative (30-day) results. J Vasc Surg 2002; 35(1): 125–130.

317. Ferguson GG. Extracranial carotid artery surgery. Clin Neurosurg 1982; 29:543–574.

318. Poisik A, et al. The safety and efficacy of fixed dosing heparin in carotid endarterectomy. Neurosurgery 1999; 45:434–442.

319. Chandler W, Ercius M, Ford J. The effect of heparin reversal after carotid endarterectomy. J Neurosurg 1982; 56:97–102.

320. Mauney M, et al. Stroke rate is markedly reduced after carotid endarterectomy by avoidance of protamine. J Vasc Surg 1995; 22(3): 264–270.

321. Safar HA, et al. Retrojugular approach for carotid endarterectomy: a prospective cohort study. J Vasc Surg 2002; 35(4): 737–740.

322. Simonian GT, et al. Mandibular subluxation for distal internal carotid exposure: technical considerations. J Vasc Surg 1999; 30(6): 1116–1120.

323. Roddy SP, et al. Factors predicting prolonged length of stay after carotid endarterectomy. J Vasc Surg 2000(32): 550–554.

324. Findlay JM. Carotid microendarterectomy. Neurosurgery 1993; 32:792–798.

325. Steiger H, Schaffler L, Liechti S. Results of microsurgical carotid endarterectomy. Acta Neurochir 1989; 100:31–38.

326. Wade J, Larson C, Hickey R. Effect of carotid endarterectomy on carotid chemoreceptor and baroreceptor function in man. N Engl J Med 1970; 282:823–829.

327. Loftus CM. Surgical management options to prevent ischemic stroke. In: Adams HP, ed. Handbook of Cerebrovascular Diseases. New York: Marcel Dekker Inc, 1993:315–358.

328. Loftus CM. Acute surgical therapeutic interventions in stroke patients. In: Selman WR, Lust WD, eds. Brain Attack: The Acute Pathophysiology of Cerebral Ischemia and Its Emergent Treatment. Philadelphia: WB Saunders, 1997.

329. Solomon R, et al. Incidence and etiology of intracerebral hemorrhage following carotid endarterectomy. J Neurosurg 1986; 64:29–34.

330. Sundt TM, Sandok BA, Whisnant JP. Carotid endarterectomy. Complications and preoperative assessment of risk. Mayo Clin Proc 1975; 50:301–306.

331. Thompson J. Complications of carotid endarterectomy and their prevention. World J Surg 1979; 3:155–165.

332. Paciaroni M, et al. Medical complications associated with carotid endarterectomy. Stroke 1999; 20:1759–1763.

333. Reed AB, et al. Preoperative risk factors for carotid endarterectomy: defining the patient at high risk. J Vasc Surg 2003; 37(6): 1191–1199.

334. Gasparis AP, et al. High-risk carotid endarterectomy: fact or fiction. J Vasc Surg 2003; 37(1): 40–46.

335. Kashyap VS, Moore WS, Quinones-Baldrich WJ. Carotid artery repair for radiation-associated atherosclerosis is a safe and durable procedure. J Vasc Surg 1999; 29(1): 90–99.

336. Kastrup A, et al. Comparison of angioplasty and stenting with cerebral protection versus endarterectomy for treatment of internal carotid stenosis in elderly patients. J Vasc Surg 2004; 40:945–951.

337. Hobson RW, et al. Carotid artery stenting is associated with increased complications in octogenarians: 30-day stroke and death rates in the CREST lead-in phase. J Vasc Surg 2004; 40:1106–1111.

338. Alamowitch S, et al. Risk, causes, and prevention of ischaemic stroke in elderly patients with symptomatic internal-carotid-artery stenosis. Lancet 2001; 357:1154–1160.

339. Matsumoto G, Cossman D, Callow A. Hazards and safeguards during carotid endarterectomy. Technical considerations. Am J Surg 1977; 133:458–462.

340. Riles T, Kopelman I, Imparato A. Myocardial infarction following carotid endarterectomy: a review of 683 operations. Surgery 1979; 859:249–252.

341. Wylie E, Ehrenfeld W. Extracranial Occlusive Cerebrovascular Disease. Diagnosis and Management. Philadelphia: WB Saunders, 1970.

342. Yeager R, Moneta G, McConnell D. Analysis of risk factors for myocardial infarction following carotid endarterectomy. Arch Surg 1989; 124:1142–1145.

343. Easton, J, Sherman D. Stroke and mortality rate in carotid endarterectomy: 228 consecutive operations. Stroke 1977; 8:565–568.

344. Bove E, Fry W, Gross W. Hypotension and hypertension as consequences of baroreceptor dysfunction following carotid endarterectomy. Surgery 1979; 85:633–637.

345. Tarlov E, Schmidek H, Scott R. Reflex hypotension following carotid endarterectomy: mechanism and management. J Neurosurg 1973; 39:323–327.

346. Ranson J, Imparato A, Clauss R. Factors in the mortality and morbidity associated with surgical treatment of cerebrovascular insufficiency. Circulation 1969; 269(Suppl 1): 39–40.

347. Towne J, Bernhard V. The relationship of postoperative hypertension to complications following carotid endarterectomy. Surgery 1980; 88:575–580.

348. Ouriel K, et al. Intracerebral hemorrhage after carotid endarterectomy: incidence, contribution to neurologic morbidity, and predictive factors. J Vasc Surg 1999; 29(1): 82–89.

349. Hosoda K, et al. Cerebral vasoreactivity and internal carotid artery flow help to identify patients at risk for hyperperfusion after carotid endarterectomy. Stroke 2001; 32:1567–1582.

350. McCabe DHJ, Brown MM, Clifton A. Fatal cerebral reperfusion hemorrhage after carotid stenting. Stroke 1999; 30:2483–2486.

351. Radak D, et al. Immediate reoperation for perioperative stroke after 2250 carotid endarterectomies: differences between intraoperative and early postoperative stroke. J Vasc Surg 1999; 30(2): 245–251.

352. Hertzer N, Feldman B, Tucker H. A prospective study of the incidence of injury to the craniat nerves during carotid endarterectomy. Surg Gynecol Obstet 1980; 151:781–784.

353. Dunsker S. Complications of carotid endarterectomy. Clin Neurosurg 1976; 23:336–341.

354. Ehrenfeld W, Hays R. False aneurysm after carotid endarterectomy. Arch Surg 1972; 104:288–291.

355. Smith R, Perdue G, Collier R. Post-operative false aneurysm of the carotid artery. Am Surg 1970; 36:335–341.

356. Sheehan MK, et al. Timing of postcarotid complications: a guide to safe discharge planning. J Vasc Surg 2001; 34(1): 13–16.

357. Dietrich E, Ndiaye M, Reid D. Stenting in the carotid artery: initial experience in 110 patients. J Endovasc Surg 1996; 3:42–62.

358. Theron JG, Payelle GG, Coskun O, Huet HF, Guimaraens L. Carotid stenosis: Treatment with protected balloon angioplasty and stent placement. Radiology. 1996; 201:627–636.

359. Yadav JS, Roubin GS, Iyer S, et al. Elective stenting of the extracranial carotid arteries. Circulation 1997; 95:376–381.

360. Guterman L, Hopkins L. American Association of Neurological Surgeons. Philadelphia, 1998.

361. Rosenwasser R, Shanno G. Angioplasty and stenting for carotid atherosclerotic disease. Neurosurg Clin North Am 2000; 11:323–330.
362. Lanzino G, Mericle RA, Lopes DK, Wahkloo AK, Guterman LR, Hopkins LN. Percutaneous transluminal angioplasty and stent placement for recurrent carotid artery stenosis. J Neurosurg 1999; 90:688–694.
363. Naylor AR, Bolia A, Abbott RJ, et al. Randomized study of carotid angioplasty and stenting versus carotid endarterectomy: A stopped trial. J Vasc Surg 1998;28:326–334.
364. Alberts M. Results of a multicenter prospective randomized trial of carotid artery stenting versus carotid endarterectomy. Stroke 2001; 32:325.
365. Hasso AN, Bird CR, Zinke DE, Thompson JR, Fibromuscular dysplasia of the internal carotid artery: Percutaneous transluminal angioplasty. AM J Radiol 1980; 136:956–960.

CHAPTER 2

Radiographic Studies

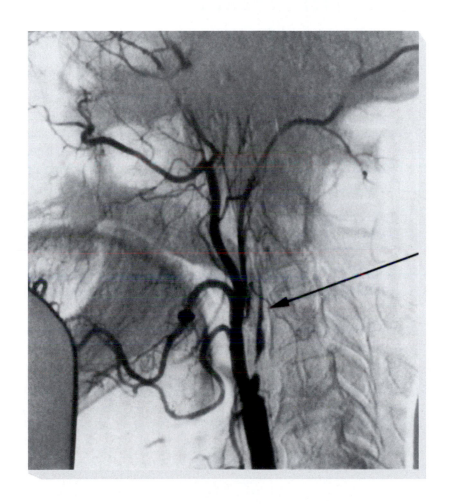

2-1

Low Bifurcation of the Carotid Artery with Symptomatic Plaque Just at the Origin of the Internal Carotid Artery

AP (A) and lateral (B) radiographs of common carotid injection are shown. In this case the carotid bifurcation is just in front of the body of the C5 vertebra and the plaque does not ascend higher than the C4-5 disc space. Difficulties can arise with an exposure at this low level, where the carotid artery dives deep to the sternocleidomastoid and omohyoid muscles. Anatomic structures that will be encountered and probably divided include the omohyoid muscle (see Figs. 3-20 and 3-21) and some accessory branches from the jugular vein that are similar to the common facial vein but about three inches lower in anatomic location (Fig. 3-12). The difficulties with a low bifurcation of this type are: (i) securing enough exposure of the common carotid artery (CCA) to ensure adequate placement of the Rummel tourniquet and (ii) cross-clamping below that site in case placement of an indwelling shunt is needed. In the AP view (A), the internal carotid artery (ICA) swings laterally and thus a standard operating position will suffice. No unusual degree of head turning is required to adequately expose the ICA in this case.

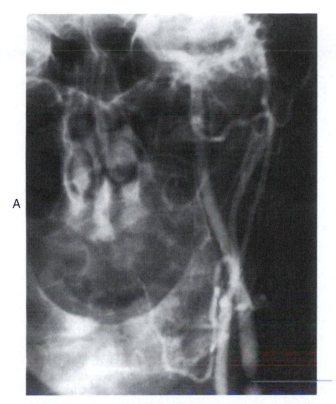

Area of stenosis
in ICA

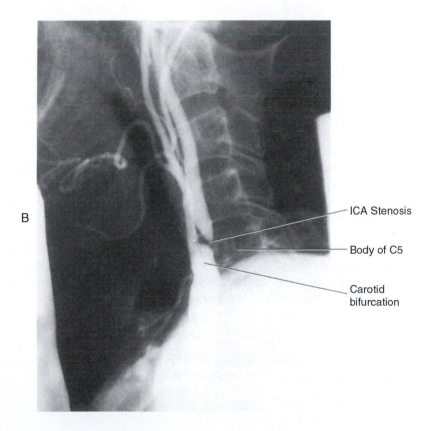

ICA Stenosis

Body of C5

Carotid
bifurcation

2-2

High Bifurcation of the Cervical Carotid Artery

These lateral radiographs (A, conventional; B, subtracted; C, digital) of a CCA injection demonstrate what I consider to be a relatively high bifurcation and high extension of the plaque into the ICA. Two major landmarks give some clue as to the degree of difficulty of the high exposure, although it is never possible to determine with certainty just how high the surgical exposure will need to extend. The first of these landmarks is the angle of the mandible, which can be palpated and marked before the skin incision (A), thereby giving some clue as to the degree of difficulty that will be encountered in the exposure. The second anatomic landmark is the position of both the bifurcation and the distal extent of the ICA plaque in relation to the cervical section of the spine. In this case, the bifurcation is at the level of the body of C2, and the ICA will need to be exposed at about the C1-2 junction. As emphasized elsewhere in this text, the cardinal principle regarding the ICA is that control must be obtained well distal to the top of the plaque before any consideration of ICA cross-clamping. Failure to do this could result in either embolization of material from cross-clamping or the inability to place a shunt above the area of atheroma, with possible particulate embolization during insertion of the shunt.

A number of surgical strategies must be used when a high bifurcation is encountered, and they will be discussed in greater detail elsewhere in the book (Figs. 3-23 to 3-25). My basic philosophy is that the surgeon needs to be prepared for a high exposure in essentially every carotid surgical procedure. It is far simpler to have the carotid artery well exposed from the beginning than trying either to work up a dark tunnel or to go back and recreate the exposure in the middle of the procedure. The skin incision thus goes high and behind the ear in nearly every case (Fig. 3-5), and the anterior border of the sternocleidomastoid muscle is dissected to expose the high jugular vein (Figs. 3-24 and 3-25). A plane of dissection is developed between the jugular vein and the ICA. In an exposure as high as the one illustrated here, the hypoglossal nerve will be mobilized (Fig. 3-22) and the digastric muscle most likely will be at least partially transected (Fig. 3-24). The use of the hinged retractor is particularly important in securing a well-lighted and well-exposed high exposure of the ICA.

I cannot emphasize strongly enough the importance of having the ICA properly exposed before arterial cross-clamping, possible shunting, and arterial repair. There is no worse situation in my mind than having a major electroencephalographic (EEG) change with an inadequately exposed ICA and desperate attempts to increase ICA exposure under this type of pressure.

Incidentally, it should be noted that this patient has an accessory artery (probably the ascending pharyngeal) arising from the crotch of the carotid bifurcation. It is important to identify these anomalies on preoperative angiography because failure to recognize and isolate this type of artery will result in extremely troublesome backbleeding during the arteriotomy and arterial repair. The identification of arteries such as this (which occur in my experience in approximately 5% of cases) is one of my strongest arguments in favor of conventional arteriography and against the use of magnetic resonance angiography or ultrasound alone in the preoperative evaluation of symptomatic carotid patients. (See Figs. 3-29 and 3-30.)

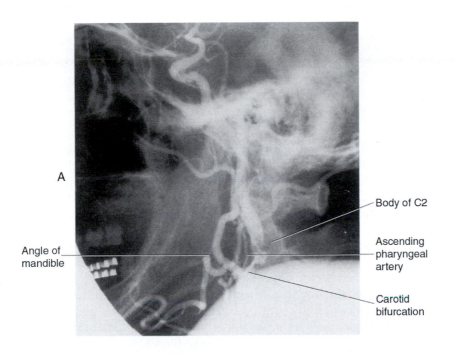

A

Angle of
mandible

Body of C2

Ascending
pharyngeal
artery

Carotid
bifurcation

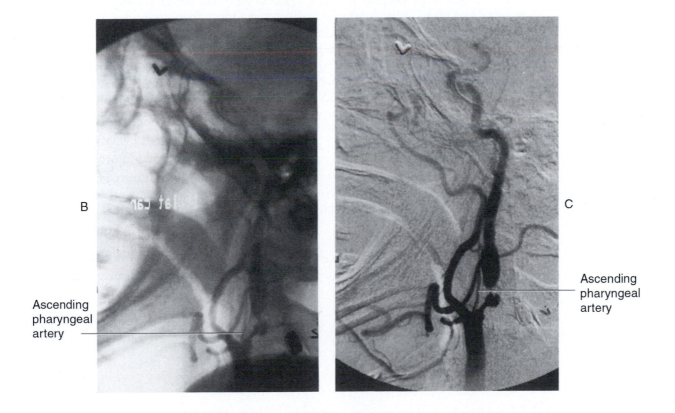

B

Ascending
pharyngeal
artery

C

Ascending
pharyngeal
artery

2-3

Side by Side

An anatomic variant that warrants special preoperative considerations is what I call the "side-by-side" carotid artery positioning, as illustrated in these AP (A) and lateral (B) views. Whereas the ICA in the AP plane usually lies directly behind the external carotid artery (ECA) or else is rotated somewhat laterally, in a side-by-side carotid artery, it swings medially and is tucked underneath the ECA as it courses medially. Invariably, there is a large kink with a lateral bend of the ICA at a somewhat higher level than is usually exposed surgically, as illustrated here by the arrow in the AP view. This type of bend can hamper shunt placement and should be recognized preoperatively.

A side-by-side carotid artery represents a more difficult anatomic dissection. In a case such as the one illustrated here, it is necessary to turn the head radically to the opposite side from the surgical incision, thereby swinging the ICA as far lateral as possible. Unfortunately, this process of head turning also brings the sternocleidomastoid muscle into such a position as to overlie the CCA and carotid bifurcation, and a much greater degree of retraction of both the sternocleidomastoid muscle and the jugular vein is necessary. I also often find it necessary to extensively mobilize the ECA in a side-by-side carotid exposure and dissect much farther around the circumference of the artery than is customarily necessary. This is done to mobilize the ECA medially and allow it to be tacked up by its adventitia if necessary. All these maneuvers are designed to pull the ICA back out from its underlying position to the point where it pops out into a more standard anatomic exposure. (See Figs. 3-4 and 3-26.)

Exposure and mobilization of the ICA must be significantly higher than the extent of the plaque, usually up to the area of the artery's lateral bend, as illustrated in the AP view by the arrow (so that the ICA essentially jumps out into a more normal position). Another strategy for accomplishing this is to tack the adventitia of the ICA laterally, once again holding it out in place for the arteriotomy.

It is tempting to consider a reverse style ICA arteriotomy—that is, leaving the side-by-side carotid artery in the position it was found and opening the ICA up its medial side rather than the customary lateral opening, although I have never had occasion to do this. Instead, I prefer to mobilize the ICA out into a more normal position and then perform the standard lateral wall common and internal carotid arteriotomy and repair.

The significance of the side-by-side carotid anatomy is that it is possible with preoperative recognition to plan positioning in such a way that a potentially difficult anatomic situation can be converted to a rather routine carotid endarterectomy.

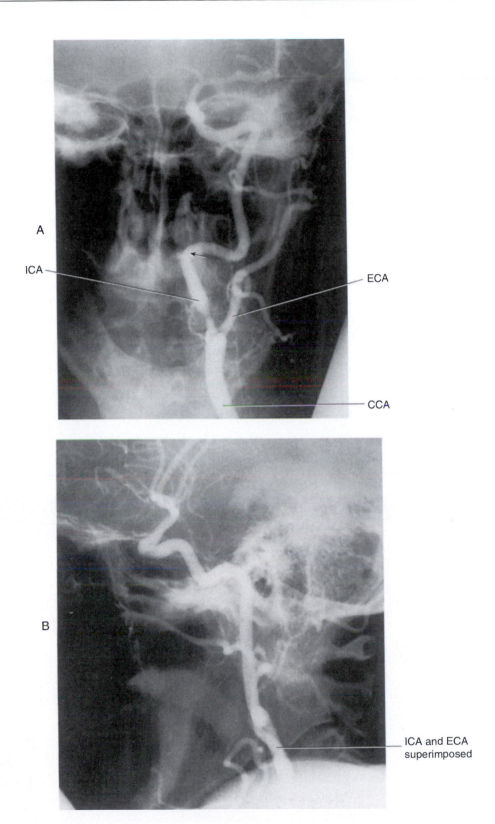

A

ICA

ECA

CCA

B

ICA and ECA
superimposed

2-4

Focal Internal Carotid Artery Ulcer

These cases illustrate the importance of relying on both the clinical history and the angiographic information in deciding which patients are appropriate surgical candidates. In this particular case, AP (A) and lateral (B) radiographs of the left CCA demonstrated a mildly stenotic lesion but with a rather punctate focal ulcer up in the ICA. The bifurcation was low, and the repair appeared to be quite simple. The patient had classic symptoms of transient ischemic attacks (TIAs) stereotypic to the appropriate artery. Shown below is a photograph of the operative specimen in the ICA, which demonstrates the pathologic correlation of a deep focal ulcer with intramural thrombus and corresponds nicely with the radiographic finding.

This type of patient and the clinical presentation illustrate to me that despite our progress with cooperative trials, there continue to be situations in which clinical judgment and the presentation of the patient will indicate that symptomatic lesions that are <50% stenotic represent appropriate surgical lesions and should be carefully considered for carotid artery reconstruction.

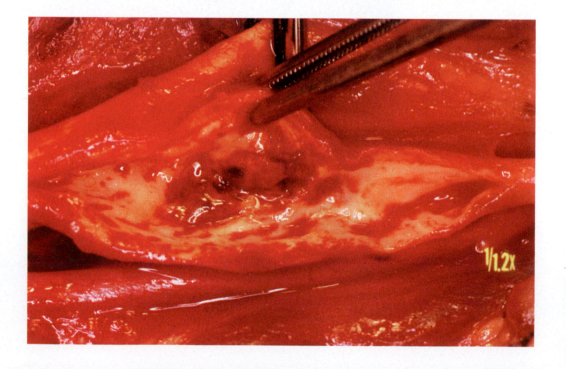

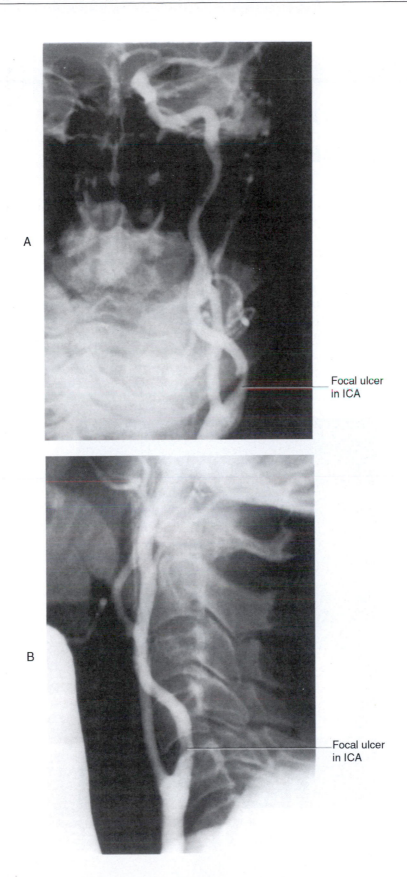

Focal ulcer
in ICA

Focal ulcer
in ICA

2-5

Deep Ulceration of a Carotid Plaque

The photographs of the AP (A) and lateral (B) CCA injection were obtained from a patient with symptomatic right carotid TIAs. Just beyond the carotid bulb, a large pooling of contrast with very little distal flow is seen yielding an initially somewhat confusing radiographic picture. Although this might be mistaken for a false or pseudoaneurysm in a patient who had undergone a previous carotid dissection, in this particular case it proved to be nothing more than an enormous, deeply ulcerated plaque with pooling of contrast material in a very deep and ragged ulcer (see pathologic specimen shown below). The straightforward surgical technique in this case entailed no unusual modifications.

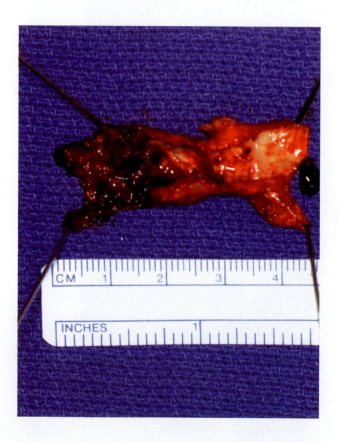

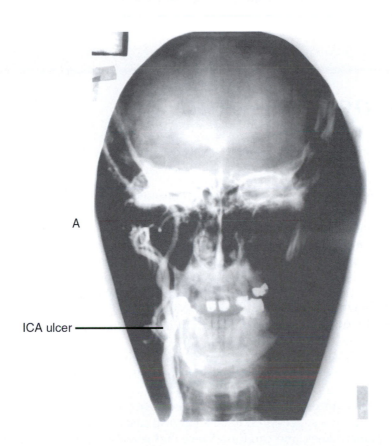

ICA ulcer ———

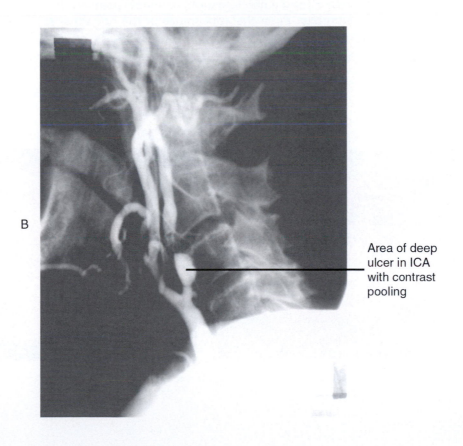

Area of deep
ulcer in ICA
with contrast
pooling

2-6

Benign Arteriogram—Bad Ulceration

These two cases illustrate again the importance of relying on the clinical history and examination in the assessment of symptomatic carotid patients. In the first case, the lateral view (A) demonstrates a double density in the ICA, but no good evidence for significant stenosis is identified. A case such as this might be passed to medical management and regarded as an insignificant carotid artery. The AP view (B) demonstrates evidence of an ulceration in the lateral wall of the carotid bulb. This particular patient had a history of TIAs refractory to medical therapy and was believed to be a surgical candidate. The operative specimen shown below (*left*) demonstrates a significant soft, friable intraluminal plaque at the carotid bulb with an ulcer as identified on the AP carotid view.

In the second case, the lateral (the AP is not available) radiograph (C) shows a jagged ulcer with minimal stenosis. The operative specimen shown below (*right*) again confirms a symptomatic ulcer.

This case demonstrates that although a casual view of the lateral arteriogram might not have suggested it to be a surgical case, careful study of the films, insistence on biplanar views, and careful reliance on the clinical history (which is clearly consistent with carotid embolic symptomatology) justified this patient's inclusion as a surgical candidate. From the appearance of the operative specimen, this was clearly the appropriate decision.

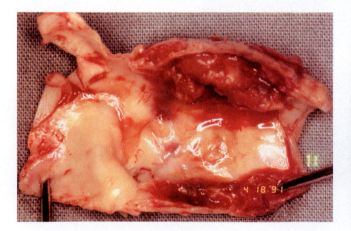

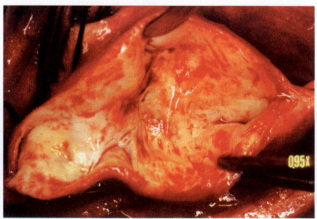

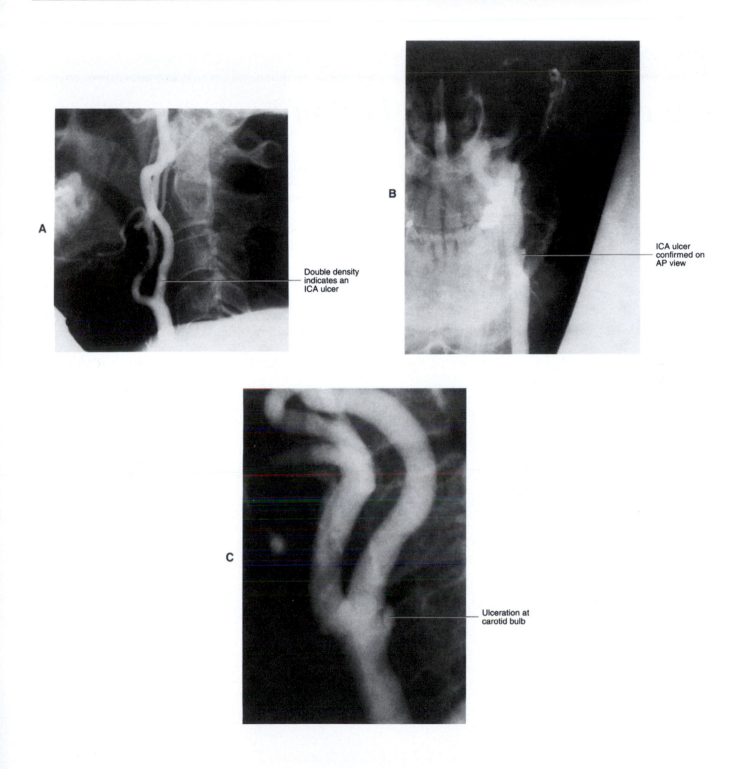

Source: From Loftus CM. Surgical management options to prevent ischemic stroke. Neurosurgery Quarterly 4(1):1–38,1994.

2-7

Ninety-Five Percent Lesion

This lateral radiograph of a CCA injection demonstrates a lesion with 95% stenosis at the takeoff of the ICA from the carotid bulb. The bifurcation is relatively low, and the plaque is not particularly extensive into the ICA. This would be considered a relatively easy arterial repair to perform.

This type of lesion is a classic representation of the lesion with >50% stenosis that the NASCET and VASST trials have proved to be best treated by surgical reconstruction of the carotid artery.

It is also an appropriate surgical lesion in asymptomatic patients according to the ACAS and ACST data.

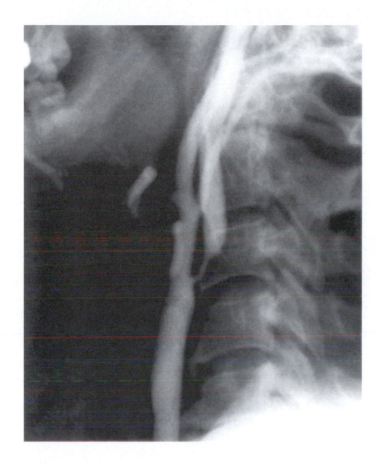

Source: From Loftus CM. Surgical management options to prevent ischemic stroke. In: Adams HP Jr, ed. Handbook of Cerebrovascular Diseases. New York: Marcel Dekker, 1993, pp. 315–358. Reprinted courtesy of Marcel Dekker, Inc.

2-8

Extensive Plaque in Common Carotid Artery with Long Arteriotomy

This lateral angiographic view of a patient with carotid TIAs demonstrates a very tight stenosis (99%) at the takeoff of the ICA and the unusual finding of a long, ulcerated plaque in the CCA as well. In my experience, this kind of CCA plaque is seldom seen except in patients who have had radiation-induced carotid vasculopathy or in reoperative cases. This patient was considered an appropriate surgical candidate. The extent of the plaque in the CCA necessitated significantly different surgical planning. The cervical incision needed to be carried much lower along the anterior border of the sternocleidomastoid muscle, essentially down to the level of the sternal notch. The operative photograph demonstrates the extent of the arteriotomy in the CCA, which engendered a long arterial suture line. The carotid reconstruction was otherwise uneventful.

In most cases of carotid endarterectomy, we go only approximately 2 cm into the CCA since the disease is customarily located at the bulb or farther distally. As will be described in Part 3: Surgical Technique, usually a sharp transection of the plaque approximately 2 cm proximal in the CCA is adequate as long as a clean transection is obtained. In a case such as this, however, I thought it was important that the ulcerations be removed wherever they could be isolated and I went as far down the CCA as was necessary until I came to a clean plane, at which point the arteriotomy was terminated.

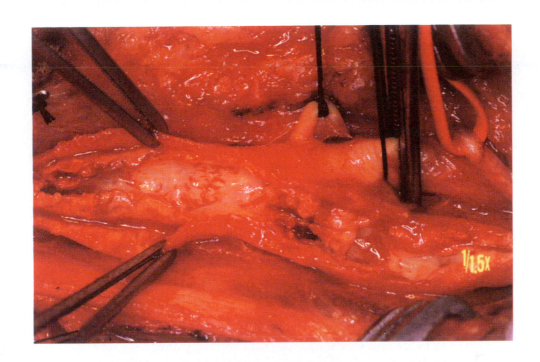

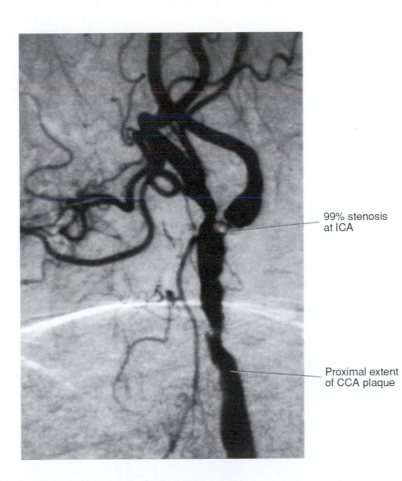

99% stenosis
at ICA

Proximal extent
of CCA plaque

2-9

String Sign

This is a most interesting and illustrative case of an error in judgment in carotid planning. This patient had a stroke referable to the ipsilateral carotid artery, and an arteriogram performed at an outside institution demonstrated what, to my mind, is a classic carotid string sign (A)—that is, a tight and almost complete stenosis at the ICA takeoff with only the very faintest reconstitution of the distal ICA and essentially no flow of contrast up into the intracranial circulation (arrow). In my estimation, this is an indication for urgent surgery. I customarily operate on a patient such as this at the earliest possible time since the propensity for complete occlusion of such a carotid artery is high, thereby lessening the possibility of reconstituting the normal carotid circulation. This is the type of patient in our clinic who undergoes full heparinization and is operated on under full heparinization.

In this particular case, the arteriogram was interpreted by an outside radiologist to be a complete carotid occlusion and the patient was sent home without any consideration of surgery. One year later, the patient presented to our clinic for consideration of a cervical laminectomy, having recovered from his stroke. At that point I reviewed the old carotid films and sent him for a duplex scan, which showed anterograde flow. His arteriogram was then repeated (B and C) and actually demonstrated a reconstitution of carotid flow with a lesion of approximately 95% stenosis but now with some flow up into the intracranial circulation. After explaining the situation to the patient, an uneventful carotid endarterectomy was performed.

It is important to recognize the carotid string sign and to insist that the angiographer obtain adequate delayed views to be certain that a putative carotid occlusion actually does not have a trace of flow warranting immediate carotid reconstruction.

A second example of a somewhat less dramatic string sign is illustrated in D and E, in which a long lesion with 99% stenosis opens up again with good distal flow up into the cranial circulation. Once again, a case such as this would be considered an urgent surgical indication in either a symptomatic or asymptomatic patient.

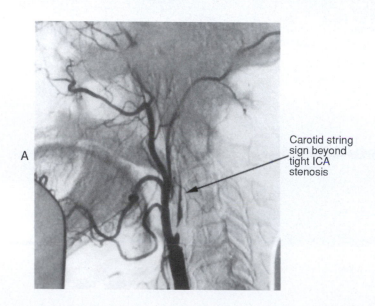

A

Carotid string
sign beyond
tight ICA
stenosis

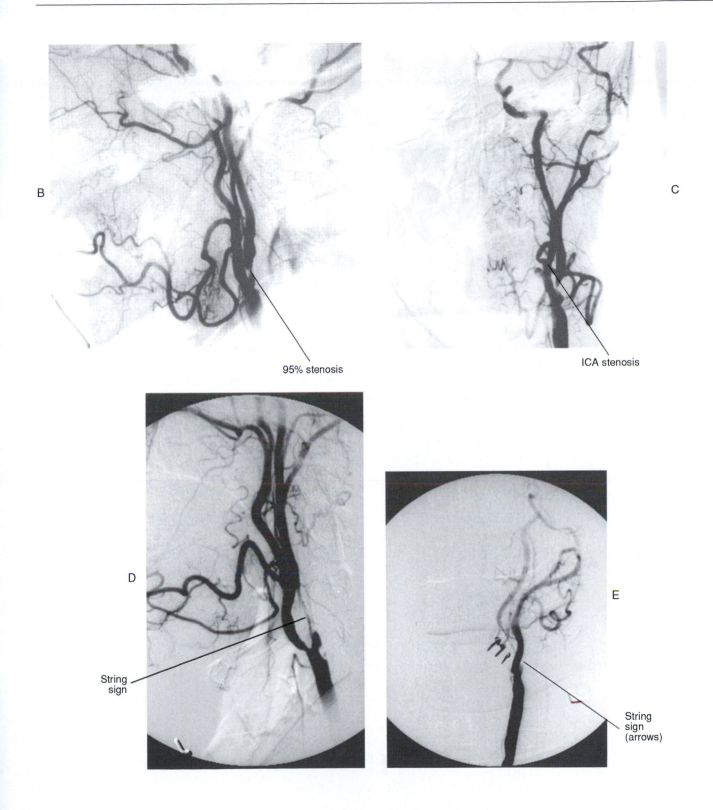

2-10

X-Ray Identification of an Ascending Pharyngeal Artery Originating at the Carotid Bifurcation

This lateral radiograph of a left carotid artery demonstrates a high bifurcation. In addition, an important anatomic anomaly is apparent, and this type of variation must be recognized before surgery. The ascending pharyngeal artery originates from the carotid bifurcation, as indicated on the photograph. If this condition is not recognized preoperatively and the vessel is not controlled in the same fashion as the superior thyroid artery, troublesome backbleeding will be the result and will render the arterial repair extremely difficult. At surgery, a vessel like this is often found to be densely adherent to either the internal or external carotid artery and it may not be immediately apparent that it is a separate vessel. However, when it is angiographically identified as it has been here, a careful search must be conducted until the vessel is identified and isolated to provide adequate hemostasis. A similar case is illustrated in an intraoperative photograph in Figs. 3-29 and 3-30.

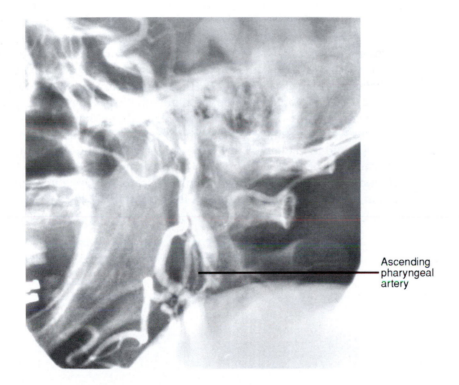

Ascending
pharyngeal
artery

2-11

Tandem Stenosis

These radiographs demonstrate bilateral AP and lateral views of a patient with carotid embolic disease, severe disease at the carotid bulbs, and tandem stenoses in the cavernous portions of the carotid artery bilaterally. In previous reports, tandem stenosis of the carotid artery has been considered a relative contraindication to cervical carotid reconstruction, the rationale being that the runoff from the cervical carotid repair would be inadequate to improve cerebral perfusion and would lead to a higher propensity for carotid thrombosis following endarterectomy. Several recent reports have disputed this (127,128) and to my knowledge current thinking suggests that tandem stenosis should not be considered a contraindication to cervical carotid repair in cases in which carotid symptomatology can be clearly localized to the cervical carotid artery. There are also reports of so-called pseudo tandem stenoses that have resolved after correction of a tight cervical carotid lesion (129). At present then, although I am interested in identifying all sites of potential cerebrovascular embolic phenomena, I do not hesitate to reconstruct the cervical carotid artery with or without the presence of tandem stenosis in patients who are otherwise believed to be appropriate surgical candidates.

On the left side (A and B), the AP view (A) shows a significant lesion just above the carotid bulb; the lateral view (B) shows a tight tandem lesion just before the carotid siphon. On the right side, the findings are similar, with a nearly occlusive carotid bulb lesion (C) and a tandem stenosis in the siphon itself (D).

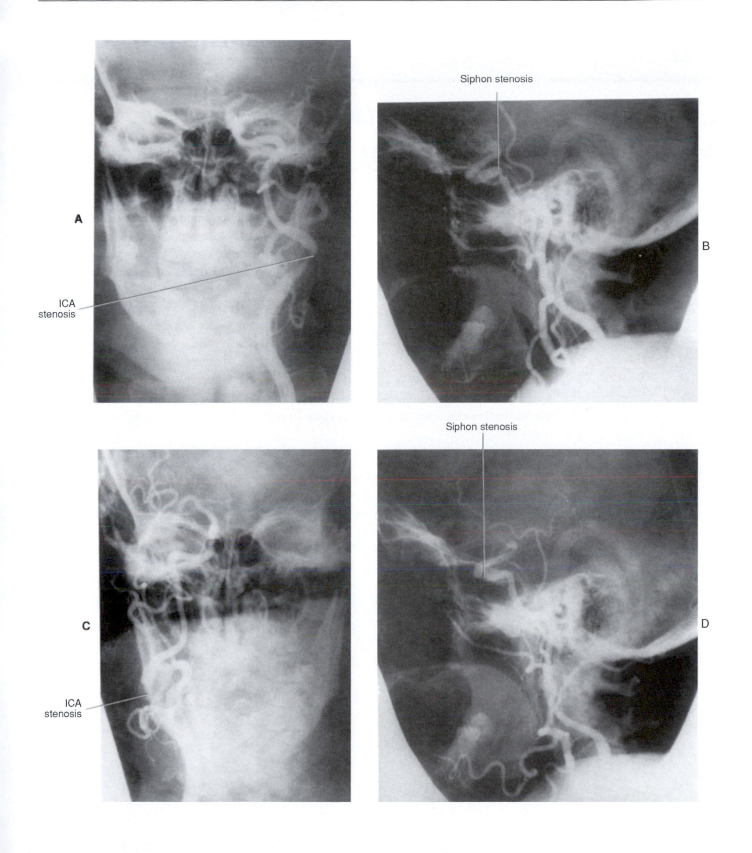

A

ICA
stenosis

Siphon stenosis

B

C

ICA
stenosis

Siphon stenosis

D

2-12

Cross Filling into Contralateral Middle Cerebral Artery

These AP radiographs (A and B) of both a left (A) and right (B) CCA injection were taken at the same time sequence following injection. The stenotic and symptomatic lesion is on the right-hand side in this patient. It can be seen that the contralateral injection fills not only the left-sided middle cerebral artery but crosses over through the anterior circulation and fills a significant portion of the right middle cerebral artery. This would indicate that the nonoperative side is clearly dominant and suggests to me that the patient is at relatively low risk during carotid endarterectomy and most likely will not require shunting.

It should be noted that I monitor the intraoperative situation identically in every case, regardless of the preoperative radiographs, and in the present era in which digital angiography and to some extent magnetic resonance angiography serve as the only preoperative studies, this kind of information may not be available. I have always found it comforting to know, however, that at the time of cross-clamping, demonstrable filling into the middle cerebral artery from the contralateral carotid artery will be available.

A similar situation exists in patients with unilateral carotid occlusion in which it can be demonstrated that the symptomatic carotid artery—the one that is to be operated on—is the dominant artery and fills both middle cerebral arteries. In this case, the need for shunting is higher and the surgical team is prepared for a greater likelihood of intraoperative monitoring changes and shunt placement. In our series, however, using monitoring-dependent shunting in every case, the shunt rate has been 15% in routine cases yet only 25% in cases of contralateral occlusion.

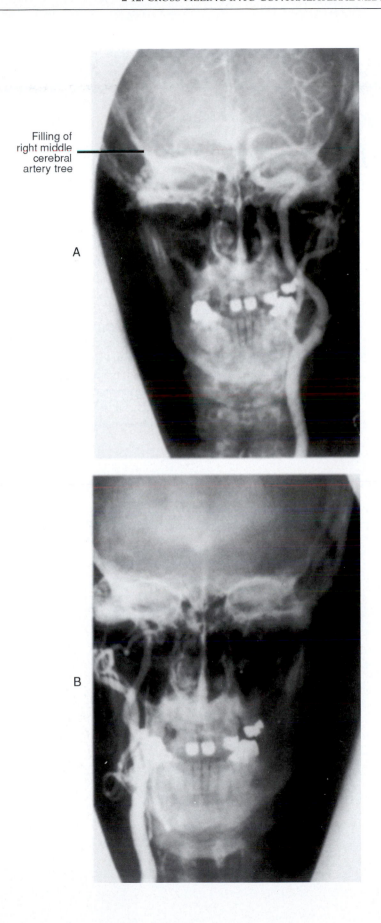

Filling of
right middle
cerebral
artery tree

A

B

2-13

Can We Predict the Need for Shunting?

This patient presented with stereotypic left carotid TIAs and had failed medical therapy. The left cervical carotid angiogram (A) demonstrates a 99% lesion, appropriate for surgery. There is also an "isolated" left MCA segment seen on the intracranial angiogram (B) which fills only from the affected left common carotid artery. The intracranial right carotid angiogram (C) shows robust filling but no crossover from right to left, presumably from a hypoplastic left A-1 segment.

My shunt rate for CEA, based on EEG criteria, is 15% of cases, increasing to 25% when contralateral occlusion is present. Clearly most patients will not require shunting, and in my experience the need for shunting cannot be reliably predicted by anatomical criteria. In this case, however, the obvious anatomical failure of collateral circulation made shunting seem more likely to us. At crossclamping the EEG changed profoundly, and a routine shunt placement was performed with a good surgical outcome.

Curiously, on this particular day, we had a visiting Japanese neurosurgeon with us observing in the OR, and his greatest desire was to see how a shunt was placed.

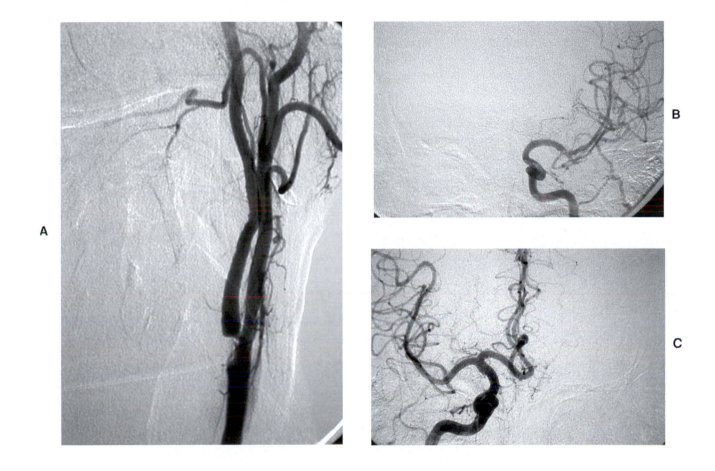

2-14

Preoperative External Carotid Artery Occlusion

These AP (A) and lateral (B) radiographs demonstrate a patient with a symptomatic stenosis of the common and internal carotid arteries and a concurrent occlusion, presumably atherosclerotic, of the ECA. At surgery, these ECAs can occasionally be reopened with removal of the plaque. Although an ECA occlusion by itself is of little consequence, it is important to recognize this variant because if it is not possible to surgically reopen the ECA, the stroke risk is somewhat increased, the reason being that at the conclusion of the surgical procedure, when the clamps are removed, there is no ECA safety valve through which air and debris can be flushed before reopening the ICA. The subject is discussed further in Part 3: Surgical Technique, in the section dealing with the sequence of clamp removal. (See Fig. 3-76.)

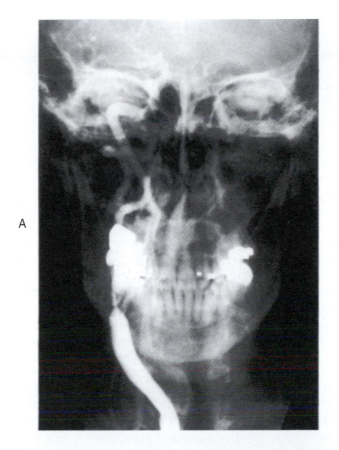

A

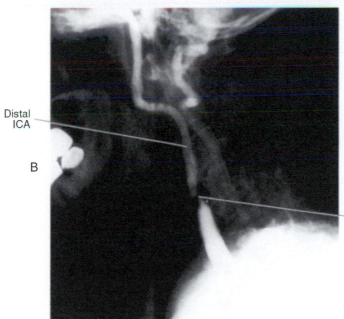

Distal
ICA

B

Focal stenosis at
carotid bulb

2-15

Internal Carotid Stump

This lateral radiograph demonstrates a CCA stenosis with occlusion of the ICA and a rather large ICA stump with a patent ECA. In patients who are having ipsilateral transient ischemic symptoms referable to ECA embolization, a stump mechanism can be implicated if several criteria are met. The theory is that thrombosis occurring within the stump yields embolization of particulate matter up the ECA, through ophthalmic collaterals and into the intracranial circulation.

There are several radiographic characteristics of a stump that support this diagnosis and point the surgeon toward consideration of a stump repair. These would include the size of the stump (greater than 1 cm), dynamic appearance of changes in stump configuration on serial arteriography, or evidence of a filling defect within the stump (indicating active thrombosis).

In this case, this patient was experiencing ischemic retinal symptoms and it was unclear whether the CCA stenosis or the stump itself was responsible. A common and external carotid endarterectomy and a stump ligation were performed, and the patient was clinically free of symptoms.

Our technique for stump repair is described later (Fig. 5-2). I do not consider it adequate to ligate the stump externally but believe instead that a formal common and external carotid endarterectomy should be performed with monitoring as usual. I have occasionally been called on to shunt the common to external carotid artery during this repair and on rare occasions have been able to reopen an ICA, which of course represents the ideal situation. I feel strongly that symptomatic carotid stumps should be explored since they represent a low-risk, simple surgical procedure with the possibility of significant benefit.

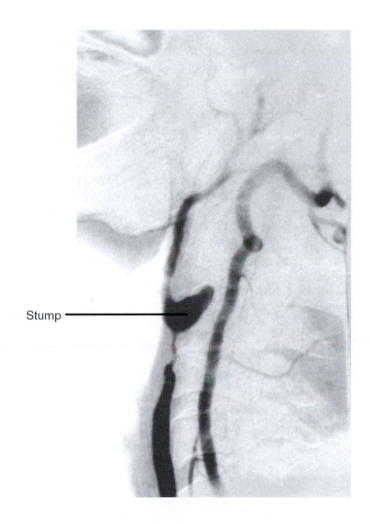

Stump

2-16

Carotid Kink

These AP (A) and lateral (B) radiographs of a CCA injection demonstrate a redundant loop or kink of the carotid artery rather high in the cervical course of the artery and well beyond the usual range of exposure for carotid endarterectomy. In my experience, redundant arterial loops of this kind have not been associated with carotid embolic symptomatology, and I have not routinely resected this type of lesion.

I have found that the primary admonition regarding carotid kinks is to be aware that a redundant vessel can form this type of kink after endarterectomy repair if circumferential dissection is done around the common and internal carotid arteries. For this reason I make every effort to dissect only the lateral and superior surfaces of the artery necessary for arterial repair except at the three points where the arteries are circumferentially isolated for arterial control. When the artery is left in its bed in this way, it is much less likely to assume a redundant coil or kink, which might interfere with the satisfactory conclusion of an arterial repair.

Please also see Figure 5-3 for the surgical strategy of repairing a large carotid kink.

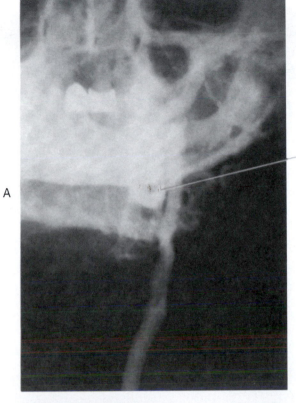

Carotid
Kink

A

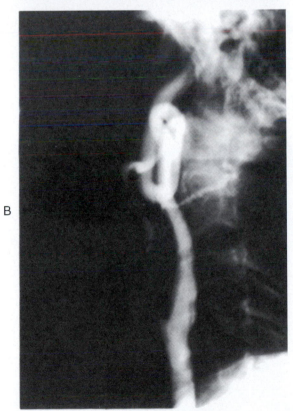

B

2-17

Carotid Stenosis with Distal Cervical Aneurysm

These AP (A) and lateral (B) views demonstrate a significant lesion at the carotid bulb and a distal aneurysm of the ICA far beyond the usual reach and exposure of carotid endarterectomy. Since this patient was clinically symptomatic and 72 years of age and because this was her dominant hemisphere, I performed a routine carotid endarterectomy and left the aneurysm untreated. In eight years of follow-up, it has caused no further problems.

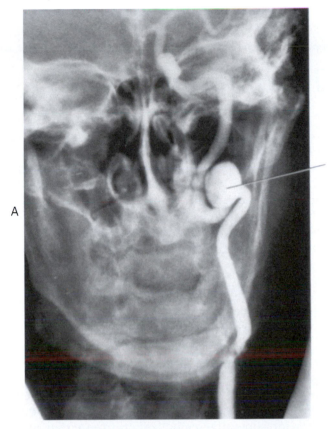

Aneurysm

A

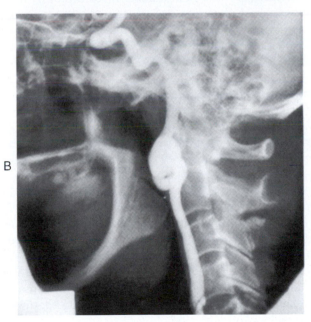

B

2-18

Intraluminal Thrombus

The problem of an intraluminal thrombus identified on arteriography in a symptomatic patient remains an area of controversy among neurovascular surgeons. In my experience, an intraluminal thrombus customarily propagates distal to an extremely tight stenosis in the ICA, as demonstrated in the two examples illustrated here. In the first (A), a single lateral radiograph demonstrates nearly complete occlusion of the ICA with a relatively low bifurcation. However, a long filling defect is seen that propagates well up into the ICA consistent with a long, tailing thrombus.

In the second case, a tight stenosis is again identified at the origin of the ICA with a much more significant filling defect that nearly obliterates the lumen of the ICA and propagates significantly higher up to the C1-2 junction (B).

The controversy concerning intraluminal thrombus centers on whether this represents a surgical emergency or whether a more conservative plan of management with anticoagulation is indicated before operative intervention. Those who advance immediate surgery believe that the risk of the patient's spontaneous embolization of this thrombus material outweighs what clearly will be higher surgical morbidity and mortality. However, a single study performed at our own institution comparing the two treatments demonstrated that a more conservative management plan was justifiable (110). It has been my concern that immediate surgery on lesions of this kind carries a high risk for intraoperative embolization from either manipulation of the vessel in preparation for cross-clamping or from the inability (shown particularly in the second case) to cross-clamp the ICA above the thrombus, thus creating the possibility of fracturing off a piece with subsequent embolization.

Because of these concerns, I have elected to manage these patients in a more conservative fashion and I immediately heparinize them and discharge them on a regimen of full warfarin anticoagulation for 6 weeks. At that point they are brought back for follow-up arteriography, which in my experience has universally demonstrated resolution of the thrombus. This is shown in the lateral radiograph of the second patient (C), in which the tight stenosis at the ICA continues to be seen but the previous filling defect and thrombus have completely resolved. At this point, a safe and uneventful carotid endarterectomy can be easily performed.

The small, nonpropagating type of intraluminal thrombus is occasionally seen just at the carotid bulb, and the presence of a small "bullet" of that type is not usually considered a contraindication to surgery in my experience. (D) is an illustration of a thrombus that does not propagate as far up the ICA and might be considered for immediate surgery. It is only the long and propagating intraluminal thrombi such as demonstrated here (and which in my experience are more common) that I manage with this conservative plan, and it has yielded good results. At the time of this writing, none of my patients on anticoagulation therapy has gone on to experience embolic phenomena during the six-weeks waiting period.

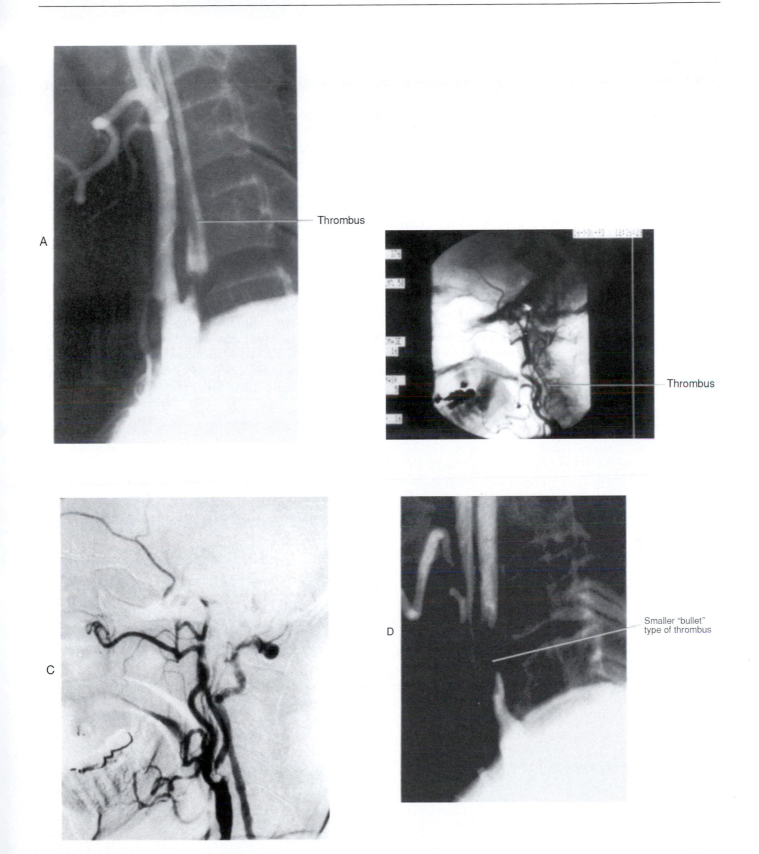

Source: From Loftus CM. Surgical management options to prevent ischemic stroke. In: Adams HP Jr, ed. Handbook of Cerebrovascular Diseases. New York: Marcel Dekker, 1993, pp. 315–358. Reprinted courtesy of Marcel Dekker, Inc.

2-19

Complication—Clot Along Suture Line

This patient had an uneventful right carotid endarterectomy. His preoperative lateral arteriogram (A) shows an approximately 60% stenotic lesion at the common and internal carotid junction. The endarterectomy procedure was totally uneventful.

Approximately 6 hours postoperatively, the patient developed a paresis of the left hand. Arteriography demonstrated a patent carotid tree but evidence of clot formation along the suture line (B). I elected to manage this patient with fulll heparinization, and within 72 hours his hand function had essentially returned to normal. I switched him from heparin to warfarin while in hospital and maintained him on anticoagulation for three months, after which time I brought him back for a follow-up arteriogram (C), which showed resolution of the clot and a technically satisfactory, nonstenotic arterial repair. The patient has remained neurologically intact since that time. Please note that this case pre-dates my use of the universal Hemashield® roof patch graft.

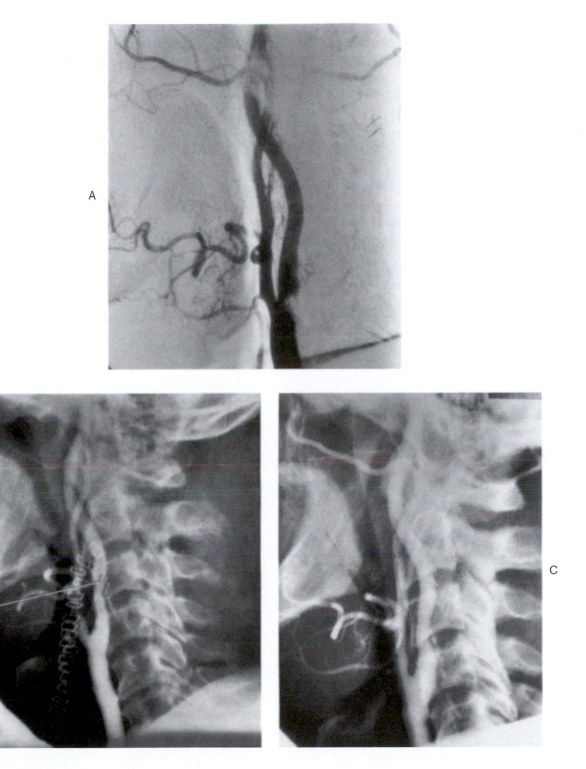

Source: From Loftus CM. Surgical management options to prevent ischemic stroke. Neurosurgery Quarterly 4(1): 1–38, 1994.

2-20

Complication—Complete Postoperative Occlusion

This patient had an uneventful carotid endarterectomy. He was also known to have a contralateral carotid occlusion. In the immediate postoperative period (approximately 1 hour after surgery), the development of a left brachial paresis was noted and the decision was made to proceed immediately to arteriography, where complete occlusion of the carotid artery was demonstrated. It is to be noted in this lateral radiograph that there is a small stump at the site of the occluded ICA and also good retrograde flow by external to internal collaterals filling the cavernous and petrous portions of the carotid artery. This retrograde flow indicates a high likelihood of the ability to reopen the vessel at surgery. This patient was immediately returned to surgery where backbleeding was quickly established on reopening the carotid tree. The carotid artery was then reconstructed with a saphenous vein patch graft, and the patient made a gratifying return to normal neurologic function.

Once again, this early case pre-dates my use of the universal Hemashield® roof patch graft.

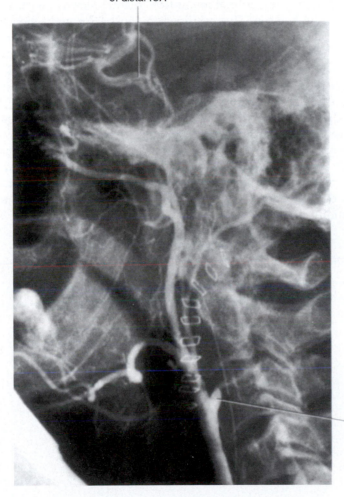

Retrograde filling
of distal ICA

Small
stump

2-21

Complication—External Carotid Artery Dissection

This single AP radiograph of a CCA injection was taken on the third postoperative day. The dilation of the arterial repair from plaque removal with a thin residual arterial wall can readily be seen. This arteriogram was performed when the patient experienced a single postoperative transient ischemic attack, and dissection of the ECA is demonstrated. This dissection is the consequence of inadequate plaque removal in the ECA at the time of arteriotomy and arterial repair. As mentioned earlier in the text, I do not hesitate at present to perform a separate ECA arteriotomy and endarterectomy when I am dissatisfied with marsupialization of the plaque from the ECA. When this is not done and a plaque remnant is left behind with a loose leading edge, an arteriogram such as this can be the consequence. Although in most cases this is a benign occurrence and has not been considered justification for reoperation, I am familiar with one case in which an ECA dissection led to thrombosis of the common and internal carotid arteries 10 days postoperatively, followed by a major and irreversible stroke. I have thus developed a very low threshold for ECA arteriotomy and repair, and this technique is illustrated in Figs. 3-57 to 3-61, 3-69 to 3-70, and 3-79.

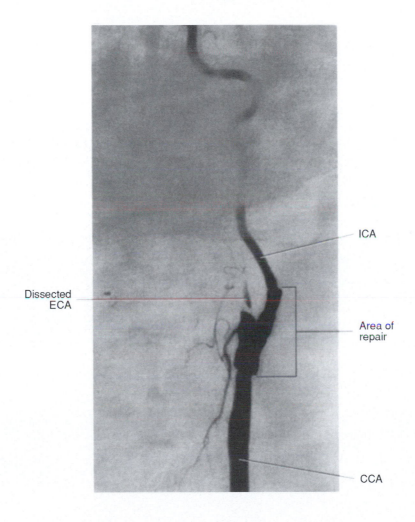

ICA

Dissected
ECA

Area of
repair

CCA

Source: From Loftus CM. Surgical management options to prevent ischemic stroke. Neurosurgery Quarterly 4(1): 1–38, 1994.

CHAPTER 3

Surgical Technique

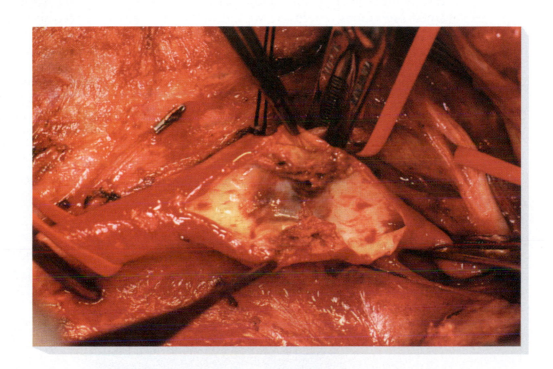

3-1

Surgical Instruments

Like most surgeons do, I have assembled for my personal use (and I treasure) a custom tray of surgical instruments specifically for carotid surgery. Some of these instruments are standard favorites, while others have been specially designed or modified by the Scanlan Company of St. Paul, Minnesota. For a number of years I have marketed, with Scanlan, the Scanlan-Loftus® carotid set, a complete set of essential instrumentation for carotid procedures (A). In (B), we illustrate specifically four Scanlan-Loftus scissors; two types of Pott's scissors to open the vessel (large and small, depending in the vessel size and degree of calcification), and also two sets of specially designed Metzenbaum-type scissors, again large and small, which I use for the dissection and exposure steps (large), and for fine work around the internal carotid or for plaque trimming in the CCA (small). In (C), I have illustrated the large and small "bulldog" clamps I use for closure of the internal and external carotid arteries. The large strong clamp occludes the ECA nicely to prevent backbleeding, while the smaller weaker clamp occludes the ICA without causing intimal damage. Finally, in (D), I show the simple Rummel-type tourniquet, handmade by the scrub nurse, which I use (with an encircling 0 silk tie) to occlude the CCA around a shunt tube if shunting is needed. If no shunt is required, the CCA is occluded throughout the case with a DeBakey-type cross-clamp only.

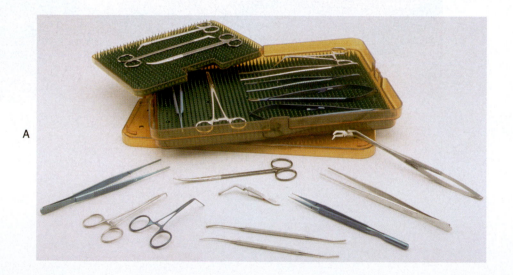

A

B

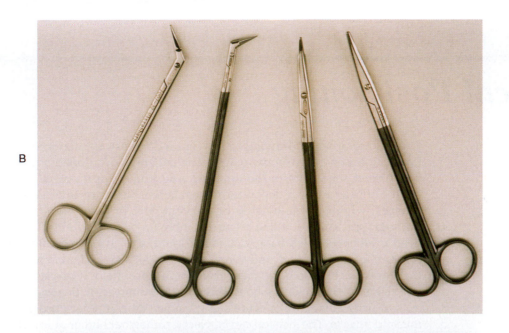

C

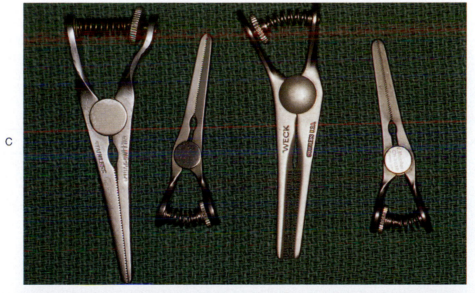

D

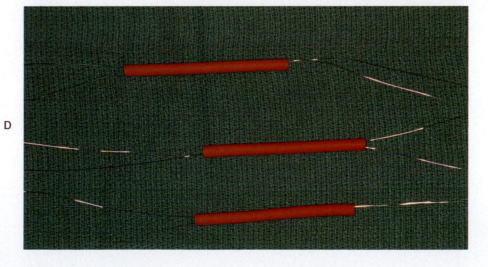

3-2

Surgical Positioning

The photograph and drawing in this figure demonstrate standard surgical positioning for a carotid endarterectomy (CEA). The patient is positioned with the head extended and turned somewhat to the opposite side from the proposed surgical incision. The degree of head turning depends on the relationship of the internal and external carotid arteries, whether side-by-side or conventional in position as outlined in Fig. 2-3, Radiographic studies, it will be turned more for a "side-by-side" carotid exposure. The head is allowed to fall back on a foam donut, and five or six folded towels or pillowcases are placed between and beneath the patient's shoulder blades, thereby permitting the shoulders to drop back, away from the surgical field. If this is not done, the surgeon will need to work over the bony shoulder prominence, which is awkward.

A vertical incision is made along the palpable anterior border of the sternocleidomastoid muscle. The incision can be placed somewhat higher or lower, depending on the height of the carotid bifurcation (Fig. 3-5). The incision can be made as low as the sternal notch or can go well up behind the ear in cases in which a high bifurcation is anticipated. The angle of the mandible as visualized on the lateral angiographic film can be drawn on the skin and thus provide some idea of the approximate position of the carotid tree in relation to surface anatomic landmarks.

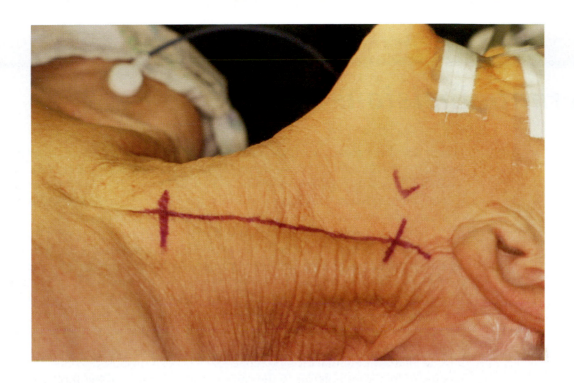

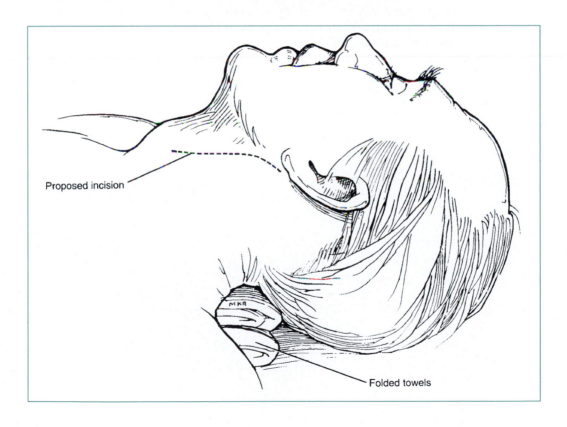

Proposed incision

Folded towels

3-3

Alternate Incisions

There are three basic incisions customarily proposed for CEA. As mentioned previously, the one I prefer is a vertical incision along the anterior border of the sternocleidomastoid muscle that tapers off behind the pinna of the ear to head toward the mastoid process. I personally find this satisfactory for high exposure in essentially every case and have never seen the need to vary this standard technique.

Some surgeons have proposed a transverse incision that fells nicely into skin creases in the anterior triangle of the neck. This is a reasonable approach; however, it entails a greater degree of difficulty to gain a high exposure, usually necessitating the use of an assistant pulling up rather heavily with army-navy retractors to expose the distal internal carotid artery (ICA) in a high case. It has been my experience that if the platysma is properly closed, there is no cosmetic difference between the vertical incision that I prefer and the transverse incision despite the fact that the latter more naturally follows the skin lines of the neck.

The third potential incision is one that has been proposed by Sundt for a very high exposure that goes anterior to the ear, up along the side of the face. For cosmetic reasons I have not considered it necessary to resort to this incision, but I do agree that it would have utility in gaining an extreme high exposure, as Sundt has so elegantly demonstrated. Likewise, in my practice I have not seen the necessity of dislocating the jaw to obtain distal ICA control.

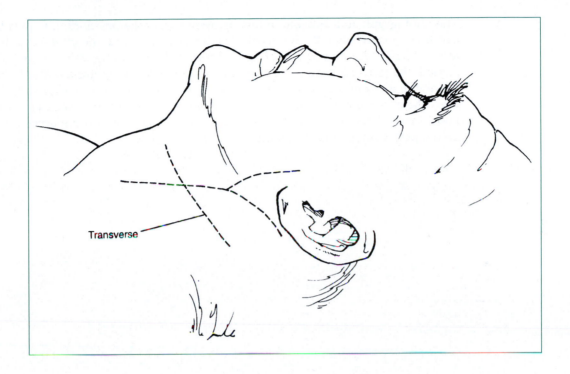

3-4

Side-by-Side Positioning

The photograph and drawing in this figure illustrate the positioning for a side-by-side carotid exposure when the ICA is hidden, tucked away underneath the external carotid artery (ECA). (An angiographic view of this is shown in Fig. 2-3.) As previously discussed, the face and head must be turned radically to the contralateral side in order to swing the ICA out into a more accessible position for this type of exposure. Even with this type of positioning, it will be necessary to do an extensive dissection along the ICA and to most likely pull it out from its adventitial bed into a more accessible position before performing endarterectomy.

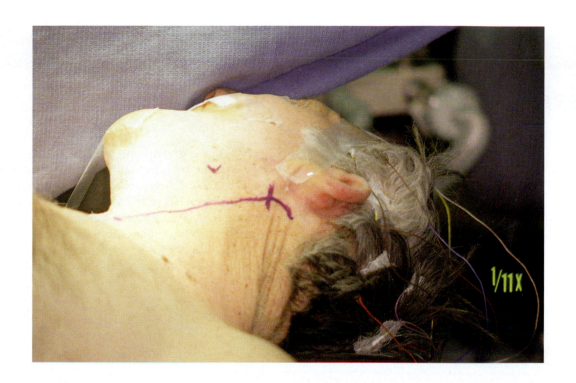

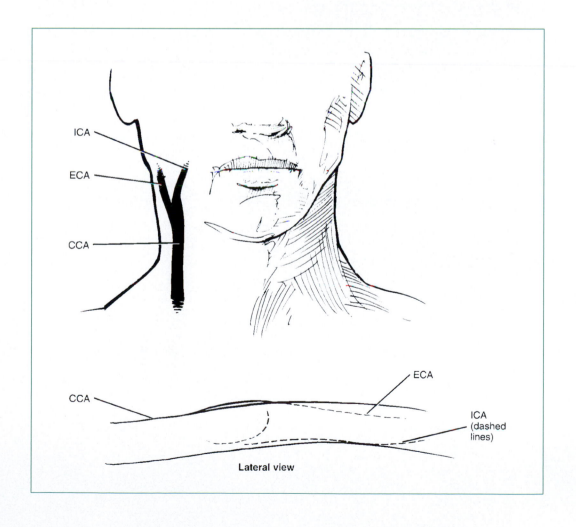

ICA

ECA

CCA

CCA

ECA

ICA (dashed lines)

Lateral view

3-5

Incision for High Bifurcation

When a high bifurcation is anticipated, I take great pains to place the incision as high as possible so that it is not necessary to come back out and extend it during the procedure. Although Sundt has suggested that the incision can be taken up in front of the ear, this leaves a scar on the face and puts the branches of the facial nerve in jeopardy. I prefer to tape the pinna of the ear back and carry the incision as high as possible beyond the angle of the jaw as it tapers posteriorly back underneath the earlobe.

In this figure, the angle of the mandible is marked and the cross hatches indicate the extent of skin incision that will be necessary to expose the carotid tree.

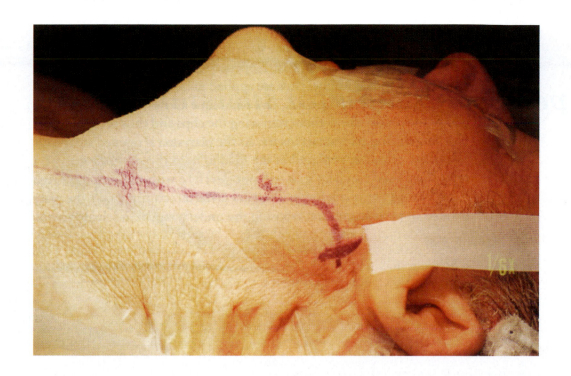

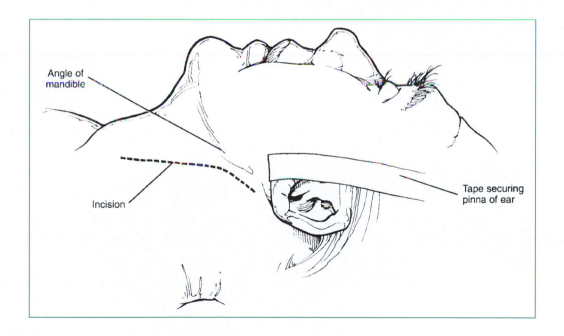

Angle of
mandible

Incision

Tape securing
pinna of ear

3-6

Draped and Ready for Incision

Following the skin prep, which is povidone-iodine only allowed to dry for five minutes, I remark the incision with a sterile marker and square off the field with four sterile towels. We then carefully apply an adhesive barrier drape, taking care not to pull the towels into the field and potentially limit the exposure. This is especially important with the towel at the cephalad end where high exposure may be needed.

The prep is gently painted-on only because of my fears that a scrubbing-type prep could dislodge friable materials from the carotid plaque and cause a stroke. Likewise I do not follow with alcohol because it smears and erases the skin markings.

In this photograph, please note the "L" shaped marking of the angle of the mandible.

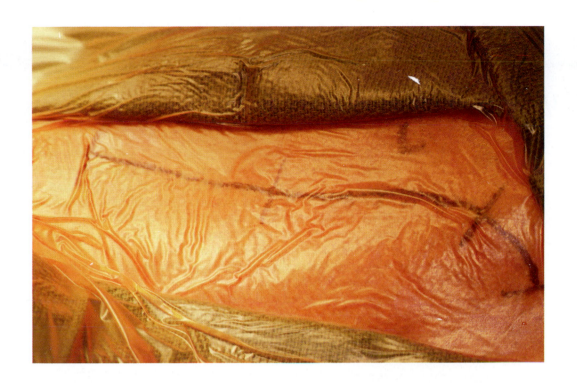

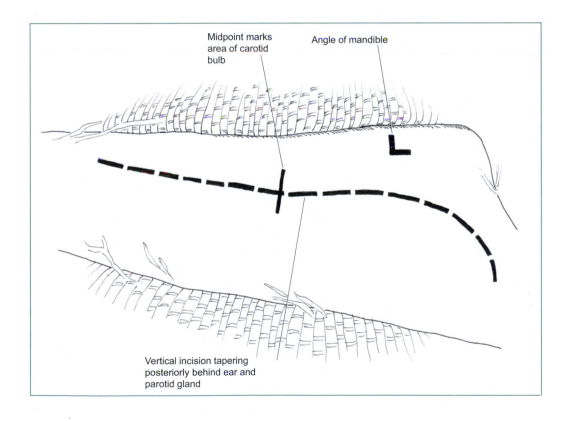

Midpoint marks
area of carotid
bulb

Angle of mandible

Vertical incision tapering
posteriorly behind ear and
parotid gland

3-7

Platysma with Michel Clips

Shown are initial stages of wound opening for CEA. I infiltrate the skin with 1% xylocaine with 1:200,000 parts of epinephrine to reduce superficial bleeding. The skin is then opened sharply down to the level of the platysma, which is left intact. Michel clips are applied to hold sponges all along the wound edge before the platysma is opened. This technique allows the platysma to be closed at the end of the procedure without removing the clips and thus prevents troublesome skin bleeding during platysmal closure. As the platysma is opened sharply, the first blunt Weitlaner retractor is placed in the field to hold the skin edges apart; the handle is typically placed caudally so it will not interfere with the surgeon's right hand.

This figure of a left-sided CEA shows the platysma sharply divided in preparation for exposing the underlying sternocleidomastoid muscle.

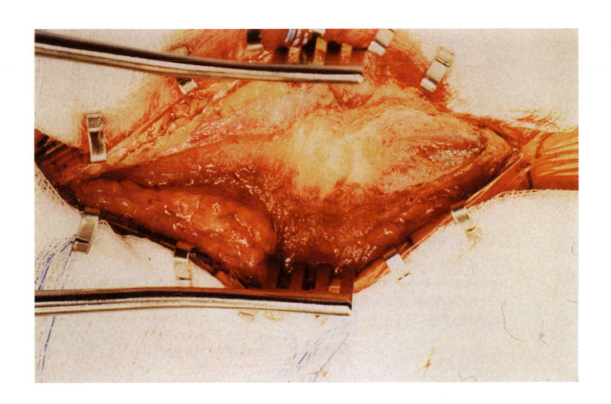

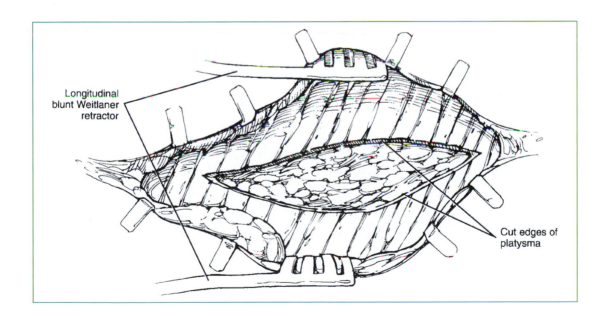

Longitudinal
blunt Weitlaner
retractor

Cut edges of
platysma

3-8

Sternocleidomastoid Muscle

Exposure of the sternocleidomastoid muscle is the key to successfully isolating both the jugular vein and carotid artery in the neck. Once the platysma has been sharply divided, a fatty layer is customarily encountered overlying the sternocleidomastoid edge. Dissection proceeds straight down along this fat until the edge of the muscle is clearly identified. There is no need to expose its entire belly, but rather the edge must be dissected out and pulled laterally. Ultimately this process exposes the jugular vein and leads to the carotid artery. At this point, a second blunt Weitlaner retractor is introduced vertically in the field to spread the incision in a caudal-cephalad direction and it also serves as a fulcrum over which the silk sutures can later be hung when the vessels are isolated. It is important to note that the first blunt Weitlaner retractor (holding the skin edges apart) may be deeply placed under both the sternocleidomastoid muscle and jugular vein on the lateral side but must be kept superficial on the medial side to avoid injury to the nerves in this region. It should be particularly noted that only *blunt* retractors are used in this area to avoid inadvertent injury to the major vessels of the neck.

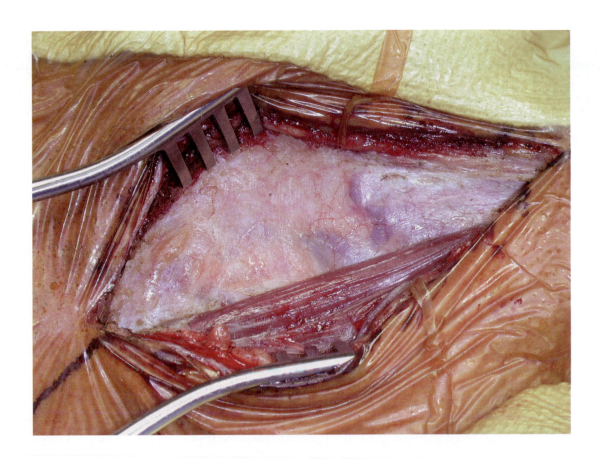

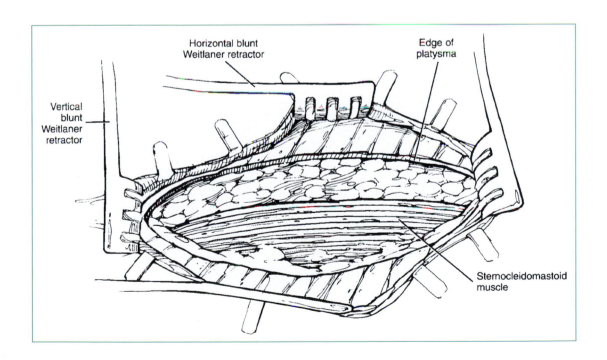

Horizontal blunt
Weitlaner retractor

Edge of
platysma

Vertical
blunt
Weitlaner
retractor

Sternocleidomastoid
muscle

3-9

Jugular Vein—Common Facial Vein

The internal jugular vein lies beneath the sternocleidomastoid muscle. As dissection proceeds in the wound and the sternocleidomastoid muscle is held back with retractor No. 1, the jugular vein comes into view. Dissection proceeds along the superficial surface of the vein until the common facial vein is identified. In every case, the common facial vein will need to be doubly ligated with 2-0 silk sutures and then divided in order to gain adequate exposure of the underlying carotid artery.

The common facial vein is first isolated by dissecting along either side of its origin with a mosquito clamp. This dissection should be done at the takeoff from the jugular vein, rather than distally. Enough facial vein must be dissected to allow placement of the silk ties and transection between them (approximately 1 cm of facial vein is needed). I prefer to ligate each end of the vein, back up these ties with medium Weck clips, and then cut between the ties and cauterize the free vein ends with the bipolar coagulator. An open vein dumps significant amounts of blood into the field and obscures the visual anatomy of the carotid tree. In this particular example, a proximal accessory unnamed branch has been ligated prior to approaching the larger common facial branch. This is a commonly seen variant.

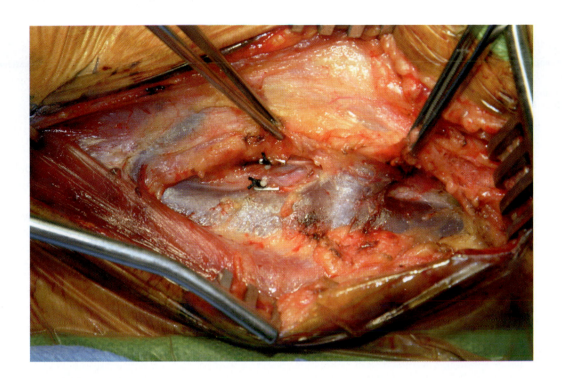

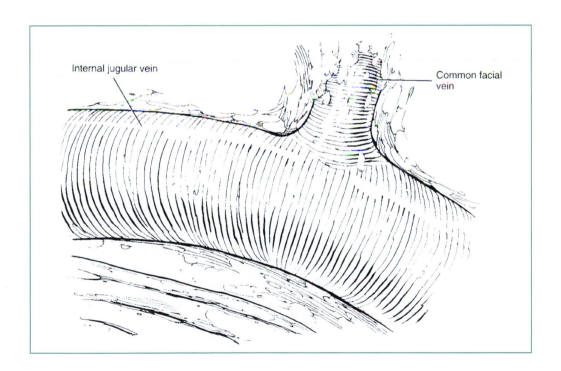

Internal jugular vein

Common facial vein

3-10

Ligation of Common Facial Vein

This figure illustrates the passage of silk ties behind the common facial vein in preparation for ligation. The right-angled mosquito clamp should pass freely behind the vein if the dissection is done properly. Any attempt to force the mosquito clamp could result in an undesirable blind tear in the back of the common facial vein.

In this figure of a left carotid exposure, three retractors are used: retractor No. 1, separating the wound edges and the lateral blade, which holds back the sternocleidomastoid muscle; retractor No. 2, widening the wound exposure in a vertical fashion; and retractor No. 3, which is a hinged Richards retractor used at the cephalad end of the wound to demonstrate the high ICA exposure, as will be seen later.

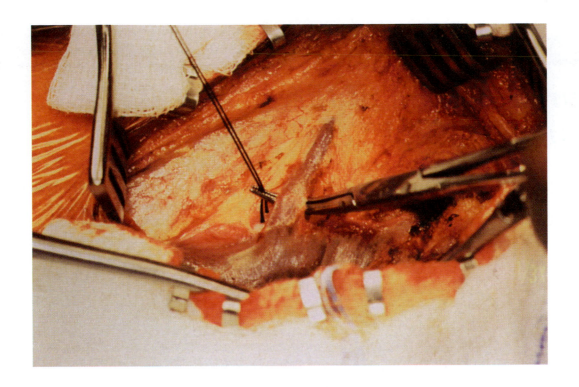

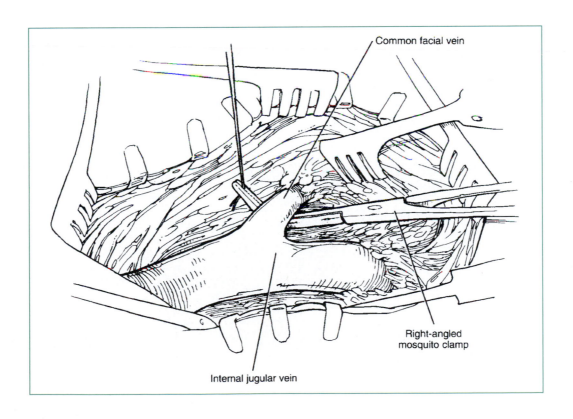

Common facial vein

Right-angled
mosquito clamp

Internal jugular vein

3-11

Secure Ligation of the Common Facial Vein

In this illustration the common facial vein has been isolated, double-ligated, and the ligatures have been backed up with medium Weck clips. The vein will now be cauterized with the bipolar before it is divided. I have often seen the silk ties work down and break away from the cut facial vein ends, and without a Weck clip backup this could cause pesky bleeding. Similarly, please note the double Weck clip strategy on each end; I have also seen single Weck clips work loose.

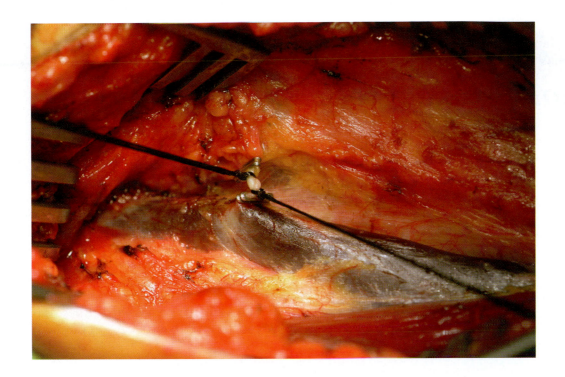

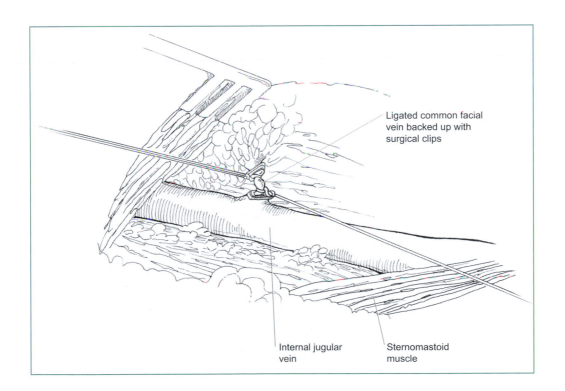

Ligated common facial
vein backed up with
surgical clips

Internal jugular
vein

Sternomastoid
muscle

3-12

Minor Branches of Facial Vein

Once the common facial vein has been ligated, clipped, and cauterized, dissection proceeds up and down the medial border of the jugular vein to open the carotid sheath and identify the underlying common carotid artery (CCA). It is particularly important at this stage to use a "no-touch" type of technique to avoid dislodging any atheromatous material from the carotid artery by harsh manipulation. I administer 5000 units of intravenous heparin as soon as the CCA is first visualized within the carotid sheath.

In this example, an accessory branch of the internal jugular vein identified at a somewhat more caudal location than the common facial vein is being doubly ligated. It is crucial to identify these branches so that they are not inadvertently torn when the jugular vein is retracted, particularly after heparin has been administered. After ligation of all of these branches, the jugular vein can be retracted if necessary with a blunt Weitlaner retractor to further expose the underlying CCA and carotid bulb.

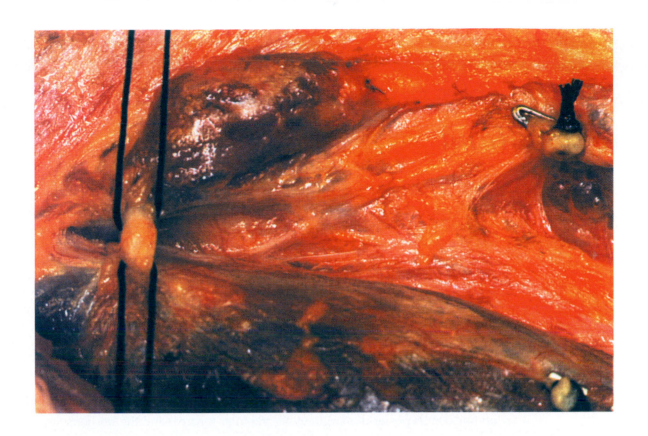

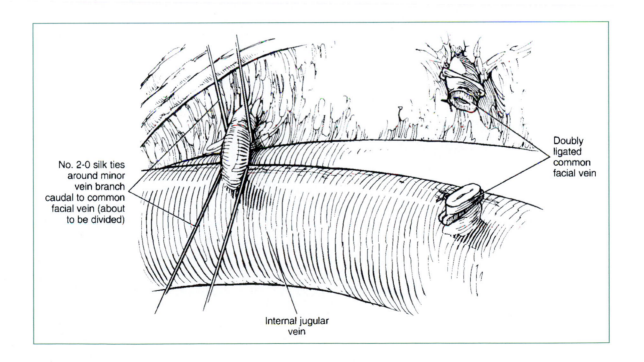

No. 2-0 silk ties around minor vein branch caudal to common facial vein (about to be divided)

Doubly ligated common facial vein

Internal jugular vein

3-13

Dissection Behind Parotid Gland

Once the platysma has been divided, it is useful to prepare the incision for a high exposure in nearly every case so that a difficult ICA repair will not necessitate returning to the superficial tissues for exposure during a critical time in the procedure. I prefer to come down the subcutaneous tissues with the electrocautery set on coagulating current; I find that this dissects down the medial sternocleidomastoid edge to the jugular vein quite nicely and hemostatically. As this is done in the cephalad end of the incision, the parotid gland will be encountered in the soft gritty tissues. I prefer to scoop behind the gland with the cautery tip, freeing it to be held forward by the hinged modified Richards retractor. This gives a nice exposure of the underlying high complex, including the jugular vein, hypoglossal nerve, and ICA as well as the digastric muscle. If the gland is transected, too much of it remains posteriorly, which obscures the view, and the risk of sialorrhea or facial nerve injury is increased.

Here the artwork demonstrates all of the anatomy in the region of the parotid gland while the photograph illustrates the plane between the gland (labeled with a (G) and held at its posterior margin by the vascular forceps) and the sternomastoid muscle. (The tendinous insertion on the mastoid process is well demonstrated here.)

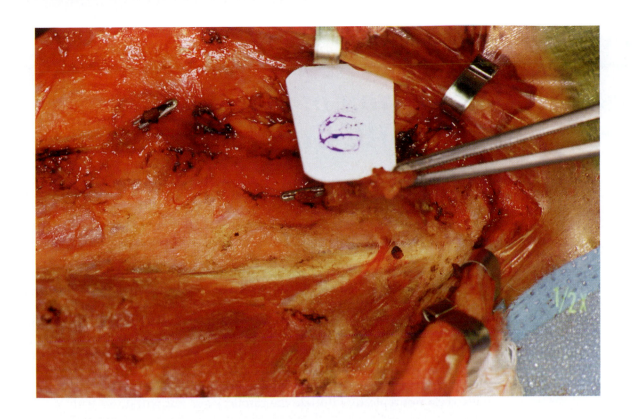

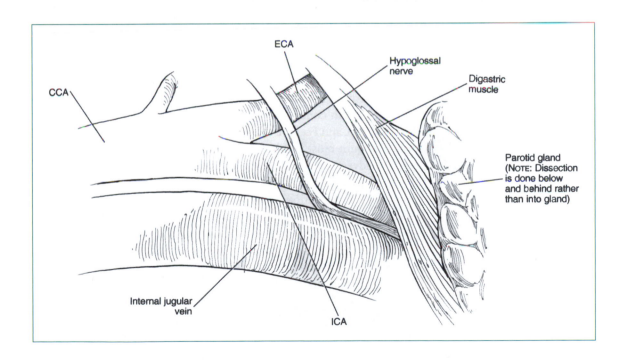

3-14

First Demonstration of Common Carotid Artery with Control

In this left CEA, the jugular vein is retracted and the carotid sheath is opened after administration of heparin to give the first exposure of the CCA. Before dissecting up into the carotid bulb and the internal and external carotid arteries, I ascertain that an adequate segment of CCA has been isolated and prepared for cross-clamping. I then establish control by passing a vessel loop around it with a right-angled mosquito clamp, and I secure this with a Rummel tourniquet, which is necessary in the event a shunt must be placed. Gaining control of the CCA at this stage ensures that any inadvertent misadventure into the carotid branches during further dissection can be quickly controlled by securing the CCA with a cross-clamp. Fortunately, however, this complication is rare. Dissection then proceeds up into the region of the carotid bulb and then up both the external and internal carotid arteries by separate incisions along the carotid sheath.

When dissecting in and about the carotid bulb, I notify the anesthesiologists in case any changes occur in blood pressure or heart rate. This is an extremely rare occurrence. I do not typically infiltrate the carotid sinus but will do so with 1% plain xylocaine if it appears that the patient's physiologic parameters are unusually susceptible to dissection of the carotid bifurcation region.

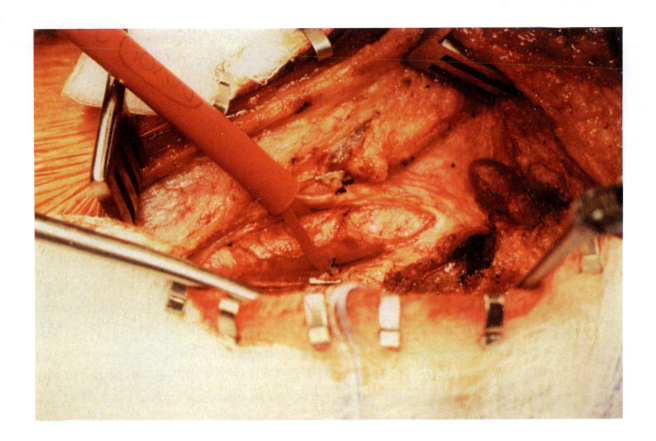

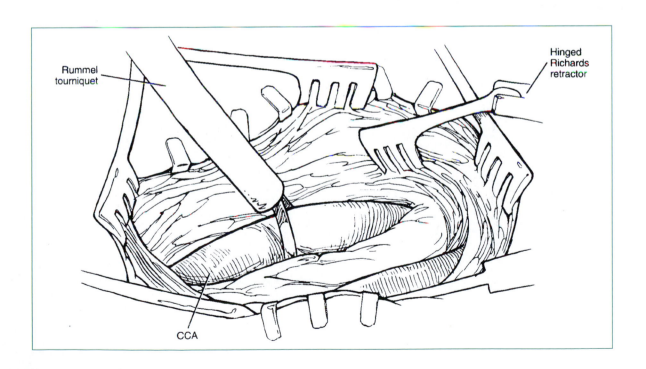

Rummel tourniquet

Hinged Richards retractor

CCA

3-15

Exposure of Carotid Artery with Retractors

This figure indicates correct placement of the three retractors necessary for adequate exposure of the carotid tree. Two blunt Weitlaner retractors are used, one oriented longitudinally with the handle directed caudally over the patient's chest. The lateral edge of this retractor is situated underneath the jugular vein and can be used directly on the vein as long as the teeth are blunt. The medial edge of this retractor is always kept under the skin superficially to prevent injury to the nerves in the anterior portion of the neck.

The second straight blunt Weitlaner retractor is used vertically as shown here to separate the rostral and caudal margins of the exposure. This is effective in retracting the superficial tissues for high exposure of the ICA. However, to adequately expose the ICA high and well above the plaque, I find it necessary to use a third hinged Richards retractor placed deep to the jugular vein laterally and in the deep tissues under the parotid gland medially. If this retractor is used gently, no palsies of the lower facial nerve branches should result. As can be seen in this figure, the hinged retractor holds apart the tissues over the distal ICA and gives a nice exposure, allowing isolation of the ICA with a silk tie well above the region of the plaque. The hinged retractor is placed early in the procedure and aids in the final dissection of the ICA.

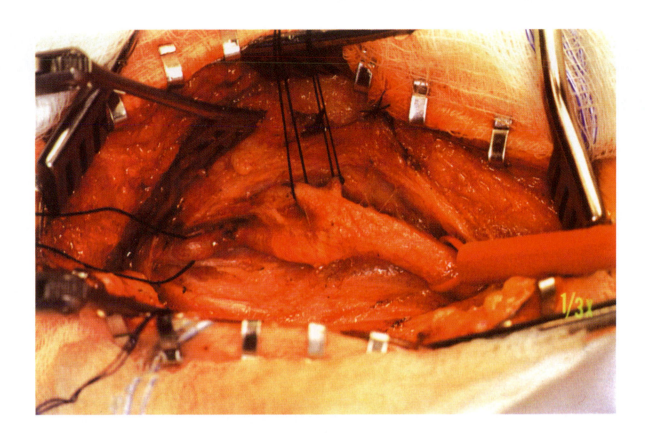

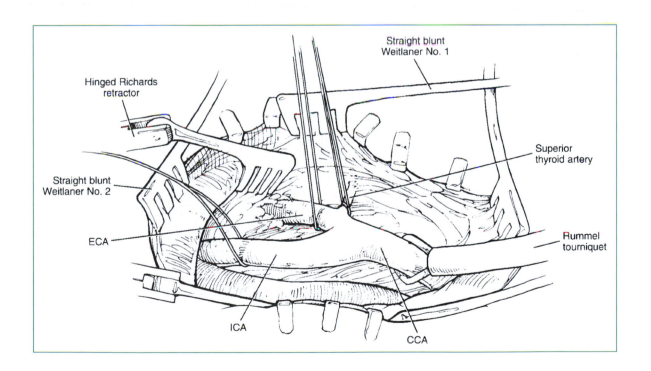

3-16

Four Sutures in the Carotid Sheath

I find it helpful to place four sutures of 4-0 silk or Neurolon in the carotid sheath, to hold open the tissue planes and elevate the carotid from its vascular bed. It is impossible to use a retractor to do this as effectively as these simple sutures. In this illustration one can see how nicely this isolates the surgical planes and defines the workspace for carotid reconstruction.

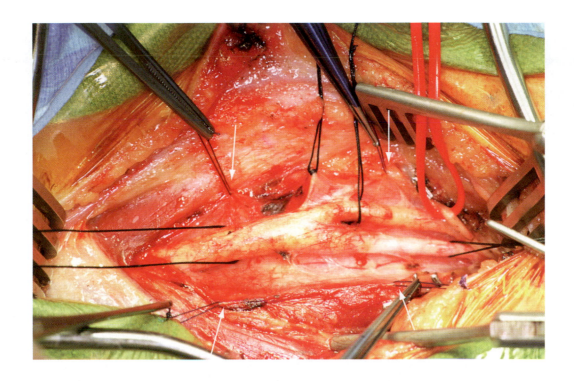

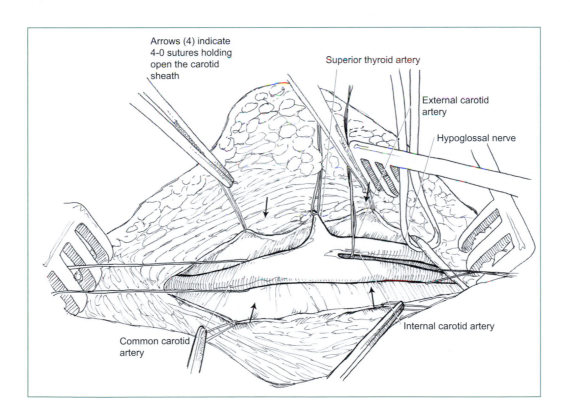

Arrows (4) indicate
4-0 sutures holding
open the carotid
sheath

Superior thyroid artery

External carotid
artery

Hypoglossal nerve

Internal carotid artery

Common carotid
artery

3-17

Unexpected Internal Carotid Artery Atresia

This patient with transient ischemic attacks was found at arteriography of the right carotid tree to have what we felt was a string sign, a narrow appearing internal carotid artery that can often be opened at exploration. The operative findings were, however, surprising and puzzling, and I have never seen such a case before or since. The common, external, and superior thyroid arteries were normal in appearance. The internal carotid was atretic, and was only a tiny string of a vessel as can be seen. I spent a fair amount of time confirming this, dissecting completely around the carotid bulb to be certain that I had not made an unwarranted anatomical assumption, but there were no other vessels. I could not design a surgical strategy to remedy this, so we simply closed the patient and recommended maximal medical therapy. He suffered no harm from the surgical exploration, fortunately.

Another curiosity of this case is that his arteriogram had shown bilateral surgical disease. Three months after this operation I explored the left carotid, which was anatomically normal (although with 80% stenosis), and a standard endarterectomy was performed on that side.

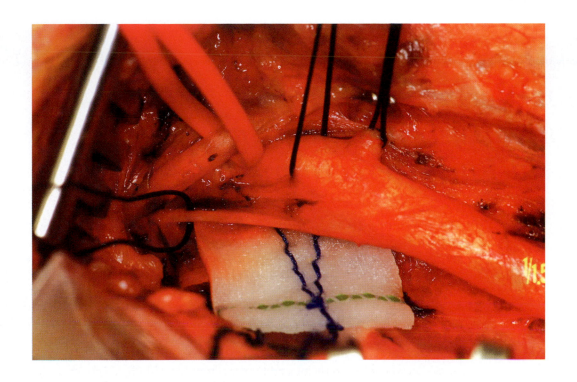

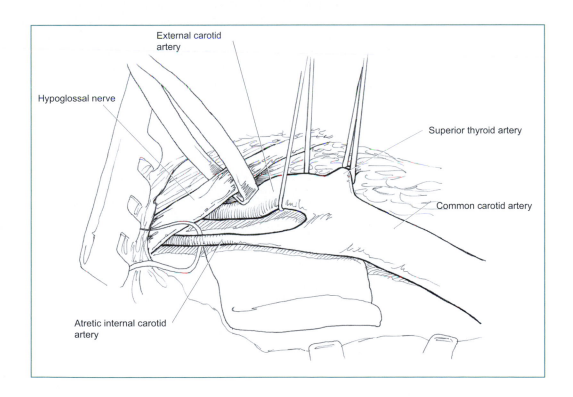

3-18

Major Nerve Structures Potentially Injured During Carotid Endarterectomy

When a carotid artery is being exposed, there are a number of nerves that are potentially vulnerable to injury through lack of anatomic knowledge. These include the hypoglossal nerve, which should be visualized in a high exposure. As mentioned elsewhere in this text, it can be isolated with the vessel loop and retracted gently from the field. The vagus nerve, which lies deep to the CCA and carotid bulb, can be injured by placement of the DeBakey cross-clamp on the proximal CCA if it is not identified. The spinal accessory nerve is very high and customarily out of the field. However, in an extremely high exposure it is conceivable that the spinal accessory nerve could be damaged and this large nerve should be readily identified. The marginal mandibular branch of the facial nerve can be injured by retraction high in the submandibular region, and it may be impossible in a high case to avoid some degree of traction injury to this nerve. However, in my experience this has been a problem that resolved spontaneously. The recurrent laryngeal nerve can be injured by injudicious placement of retractors deep on the medial exposure, and for this reason, as stated elsewhere, I always use blunt retractors and always place them just under the skin on the medial side of the exposure, whereas laterally they can be placed deep under the sternocleidomastoid muscle and under the jugular vein if necessary.

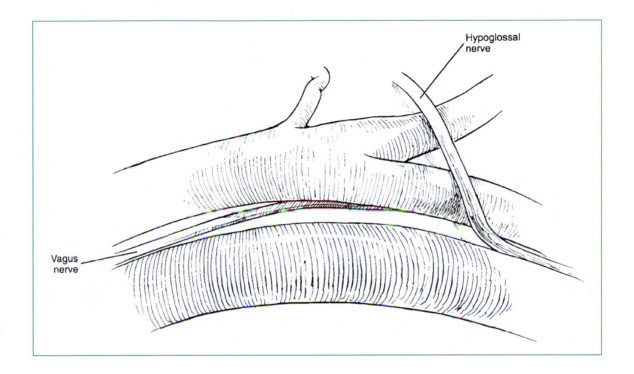

3-19

Other Nerves at Risk During Carotid Endarterectomy

The superior laryngeal and the accessory nerves are easily injured at CEA if their anatomy is unfamiliar to the surgeon. The consequences of such nerve injury are real and can be debilitating to the patient. I have illustrated here several examples of nerves which we identified, isolated, and preserved during routine carotid procedures. In (A) the superior laryngeal nerve is shown just behind the internal carotid artery in a high exposure of a left-sided CEA. This nerve can be easily injured by cautery, dissection technique, or the internal carotid cross-clamp. It is also easily preserved once the surgeon is aware of its location, which is constant in my experience.

In (B) we have illustrated a vessel loop encircling the spinal accessory nerve at a right-sided CEA. This was a case in which the dissection went a little bit far lateral and the nerve was isolated under the sternomastoid muscle. Customarily I do not dissect this far laterally.

In (C) I present a reoperative right-sided carotid case, which accounts for the scarring and the murkiness of the usual crisp tissue planes. There are two nerves isolated with vessel loops. The uppermost is the commonly seen hypoglossal nerve, which we have discussed at length. Below this, running deep to the sternomastoid muscle, we again see the accessory nerve, which we usually do not encounter. In this particular case, because of the reoperation, we dissected further lateral than usual to establish the planes and secure control, and we encountered and isolated the accessory nerve as well. Transection or traction injury of this nerve will produce a painful shoulder drop, and should be avoided, of course.

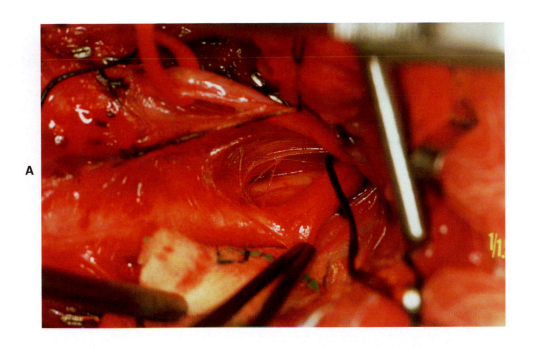

A

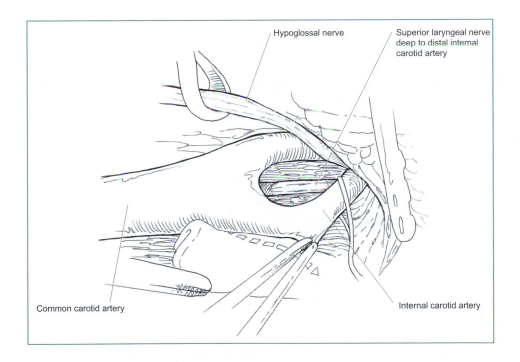

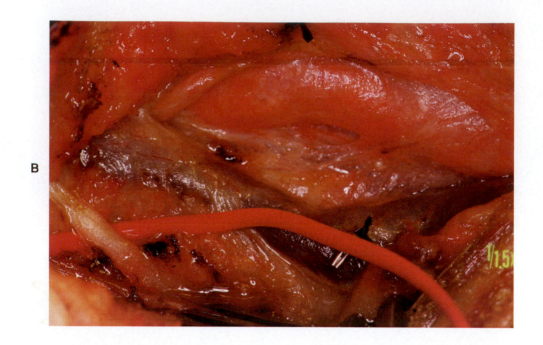

B

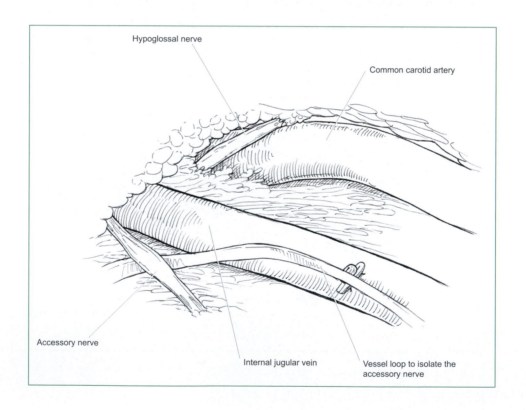

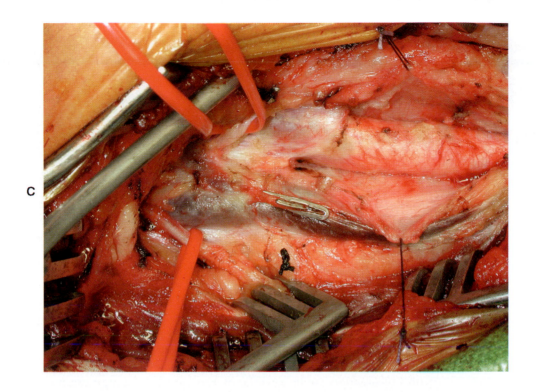

C

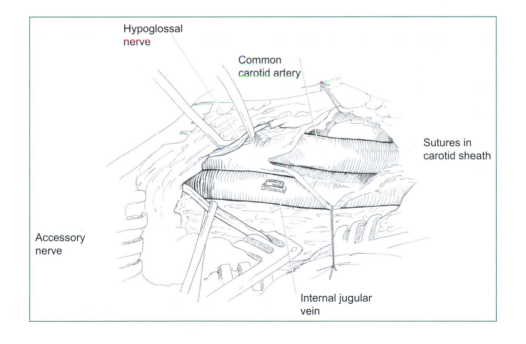

3-20

Low Bifurcation with Omohyoid Muscle

Surgery for a relatively low bifurcation of the CCA may expose the omohyoid muscle. It is crucial to establish adequate control well below the carotid bulb in case placement of a shunt is necessary. I place the DeBakey cross-clamp at least 2 cm below the encircling vessel loop so that a shunt can be placed and the vessel loop snugged down around it before the cross-clamp is removed, thereby preventing significant bleeding. In order to do this, it is often necessary to identify and either retract or transect the omohyoid muscle. The muscle can be retracted from the overlying carotid artery with the vertically placed rostral-caudal retractor or it can be cauterized with the bipolar coagulator and cut to expose an adequate length of CCA. I like to tag the two ends of the muscle with suture ligatures and re-oppose them at the conclusion of the case. The CCA dives a little more deeply at the caudal end of the wound, and a significant surface dissection is necessary to expose it. In point of fact, exposure of an extremely low carotid bifurcation can be as difficult as exposure of a high bifurcation.

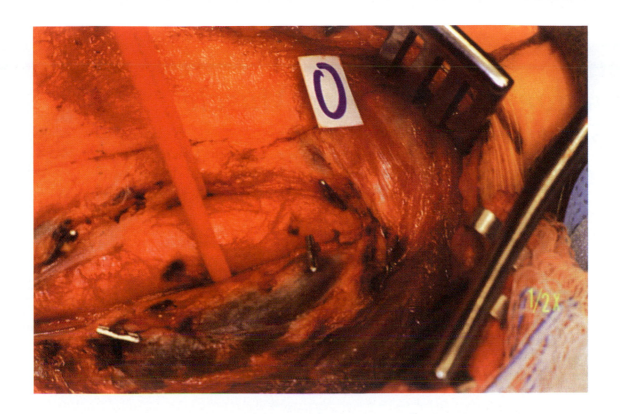

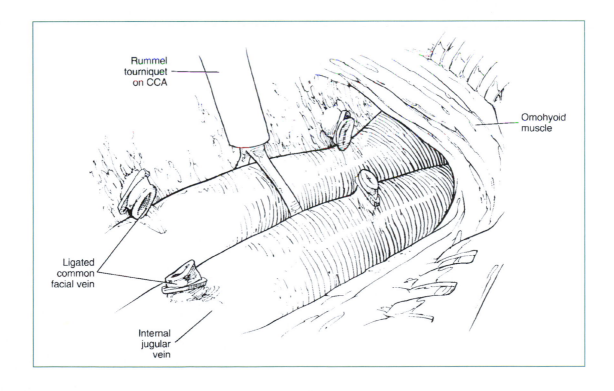

Rummel
tourniquet
on CCA

Omohyoid
muscle

Ligated
common
facial vein

Internal
jugular
vein

3-21

Division of Omohyoid Muscle to Secure Adequate Low Carotid Exposure

In this case, the bifurcation of the carotid artery is abnormally low. To obtain adequate proximal control of the carotid artery for cross-clamping, it was necessary to divide the omohyoid muscle. This is accomplished by cutting the muscle after bipolar coagulation and then placing a stitch in each end of the cut muscle. At the end of the procedure when the repair has been completed, the omohyoid muscle can be reopposed by tying these two stitches together and then introducing several more to pull the muscle together. No cosmetic or functional deformity should result from this maneuver.

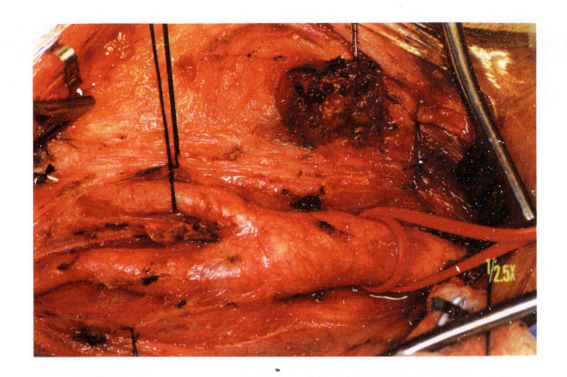

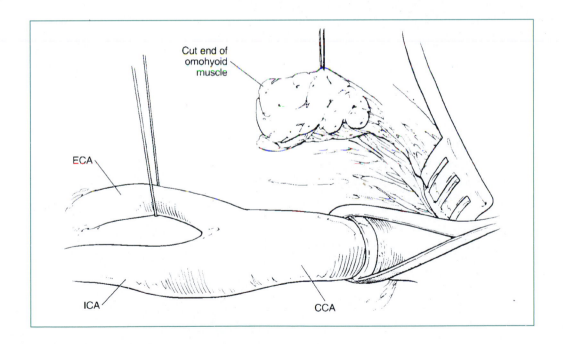

3-22

Hypoglossal Nerve

During the exposure of the ICA well above the plaque, the hypoglossal nerve is often visualized and must be dealt with. In a low bifurcation, the hypoglossal nerve may not enter the field. However, most average or high bifurcations will necessitate exposure and control of this nerve. I dissect the nerve out carefully and isolate it with a vessel loop once it is identified. When this is accomplished, even if bleeding ensues at a later point, there is no question as to the location of the nerve and inadvertent transection or cauterization of the nerve can be avoided. Only gentle retraction, if any, is applied to this nerve.

This figure shows the position of a rather straightforward hypoglossal nerve dissection. The nerve is identified as it comes down in the plane between the internal jugular vein and ICA and then loops medially over the internal and external carotid arteries, exiting to supply the tongue.

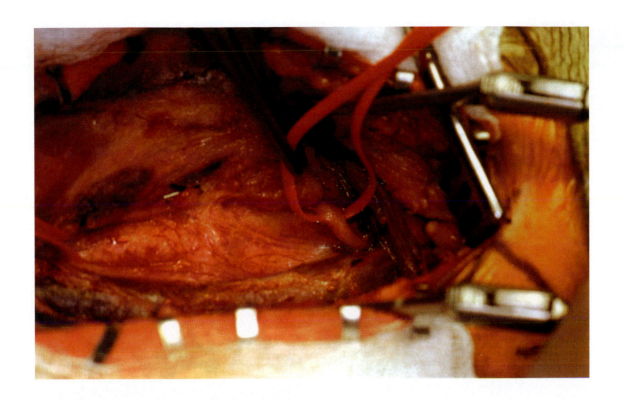

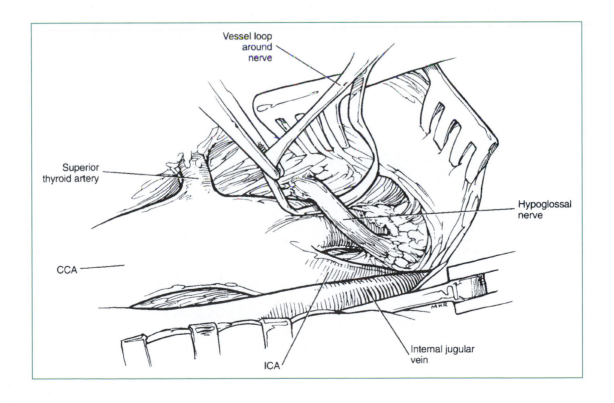

3-23

Sternomastoid Artery—An External Carotid Artery Branch

This is a right carotid endarterectomy in which there is an artery, a branch of the external carotid, intimately intertwined with the hypoglossal nerve, which has been isolated with the blue vessel loop. The digastric muscle has been cut for high exposure. This artery is called the "sternomastoid artery" by some surgeons. To achieve proper high exposure, it needs to be ligated and divided, so that the hypoglossal nerve can be further mobilized and adequate distal exposure achieved on the internal carotid artery. At the stage of the operation illustrated here, I consider the exposure to be inadequate for correct ICA control. There is, to my mind, no functional consequence to sacrifice of this minor ECA branch.

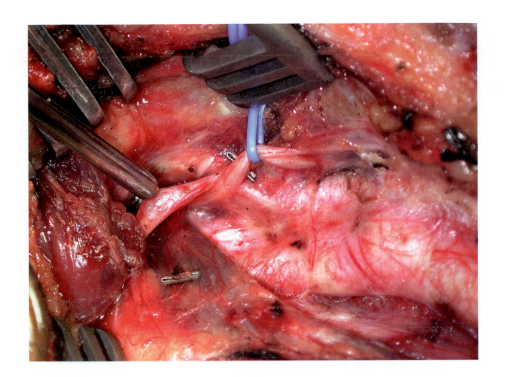

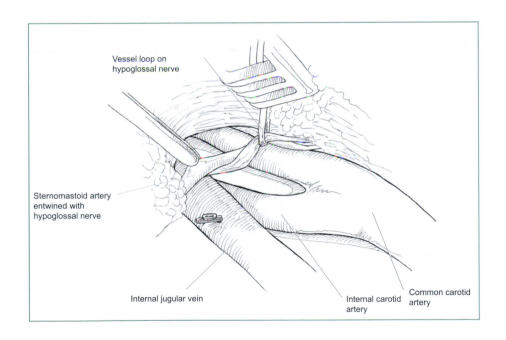

Vessel loop on
hypoglossal nerve

Sternomastoid artery
entwined with
hypoglossal nerve

Internal jugular vein

Internal carotid
artery

Common carotid
artery

3-24

High Bifurcation with Digastric Muscle and Hypoglossal Nerve—Left Carotid Exposure

Once the jugular vein has been retracted and the CCA has been isolated, the carotid sheath is opened along the midportion of the vessel to expose all branches of the carotid tree. Exposure of a high bifurcation and a high plaque in the ICA is particularly difficult and may necessitate some rather extensive dissection. I dissect along the medial border of the jugular vein while coming up the ICA. In this case, the hypoglossal nerve and ansa hypoglossi complex have been isolated with several vessel loops and it was necessary to cut the digastric muscle to obtain a high exposure of the ICA. I have found that the digastric muscle can be coagulated with bipolar cautery and transected sharply with no ill effects, and in combination with a hinged Richards retractor, this maneuver yields a very nice exposure of the distal ICA. In the photograph, a blue line has been drawn along the carotid artery in preparation for surgical incision. It should also be noted that several 4-0 silk tacking sutures were used to hold the carotid sheath open, thereby lifting the carotid bulb somewhat out of its bed and facilitating the surgical approach to the vessel.

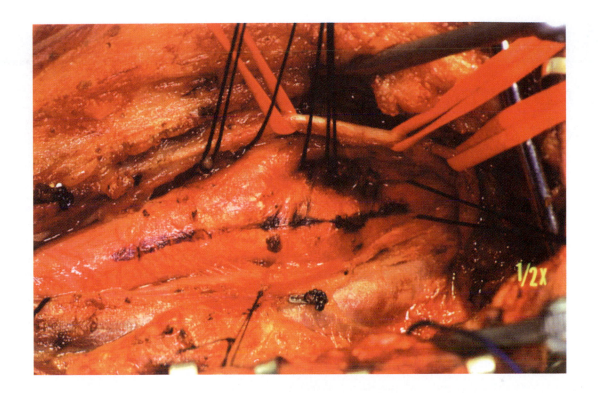

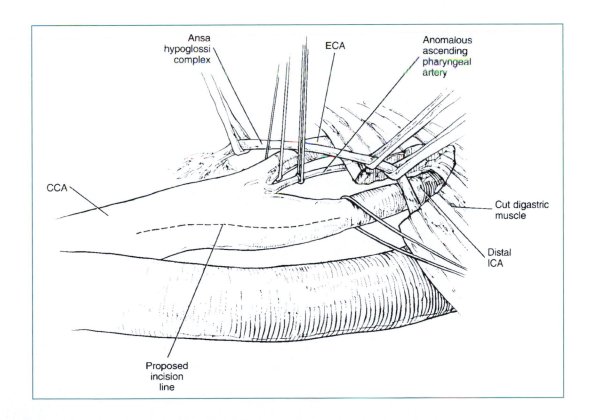

3-25

High Bifurcation with Digastric Muscle and Hypoglossal Nerve—Right Carotid Exposure

This figure is similar to the previous one except that in this case it was not necessary to cut the digastric muscle. The isolation of all branches at the carotid tree can be seen along with the vessel loop around the hypoglossal nerve and ansa hypoglossi complex.

In this case, the use of the vertical retractor to retract the top part of the digastric muscle was adequate to obtain exposure of the distal ICA.

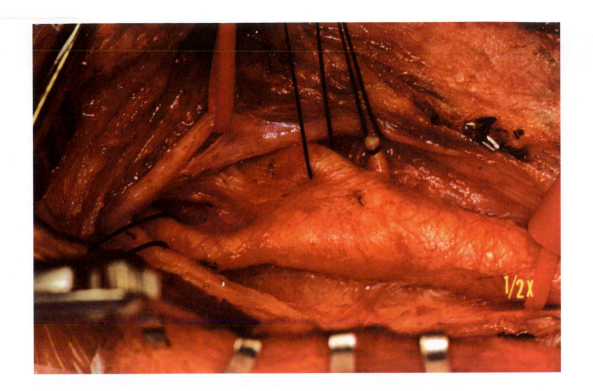

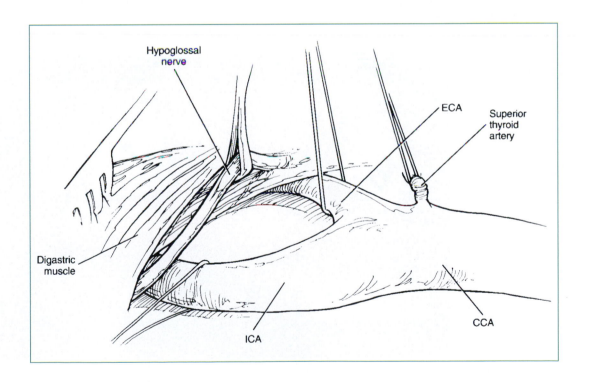

3-26

Side-by-Side Carotid Anatomy—Exposure

I have discussed the "side-by-side" rotated variation of ICA and ECA earlier in the text, and I have emphasized the special positioning of the patient needed in such a case (see Figs. 2-3 and 3-4). These two operative photographs of a right carotid exposure demonstrate the side-by-side anatomy and the risk of becoming confused if the situation is not appreciated. Before taking the pictures I marked the arteries as C, I, and E, meaning common, internal, and external carotids respectively. In (A), one can see that the internal carotid artery is medially rotated and basically out of view. By dissecting along the lateral border of the carotid tree the surgeon can deliver the ICA laterally and create a more normal anatomical picture, as has been done and illustrated in (B). The risk, of course, is that an inexperienced surgeon will mistake the ECA for the ICA, and thus do extensive dissection medial to the ECA, looking for an ICA there that will never be found. There are two ways to avoid this error: first, by understanding and expecting the variant based on the angiogram, and second, by always using the landmark of the superior thyroid artery to identify the ECA.

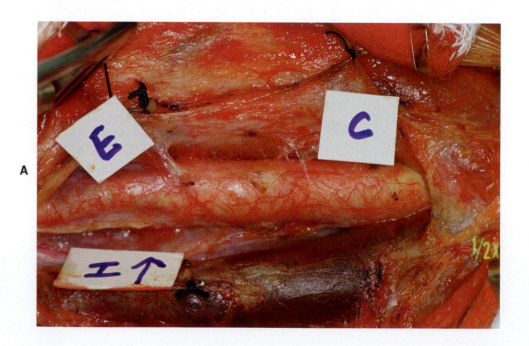

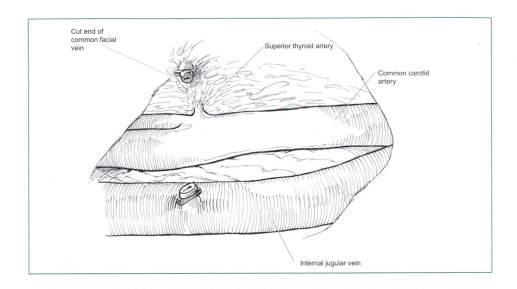

Cut end of common facial vein

Superior thyroid artery

Common carotid artery

Internal jugular vein

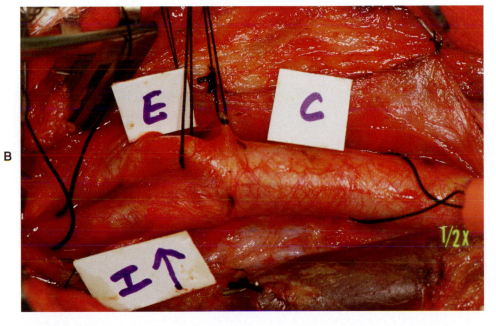

B

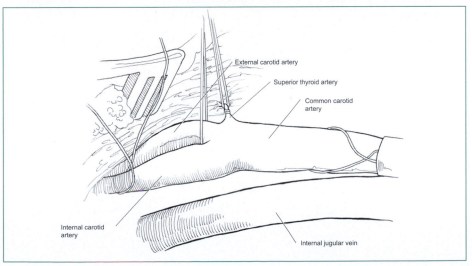

External carotid artery

Superior thyroid artery

Common carotid artery

Internal carotid artery

Internal jugular vein

3-27

Isolation of Superior Thyroid Artery—Right Carotid Exposure

A 2-0 silk looped Potts tie is placed around the superior thyroid artery to control back-bleeding. I take this tie up and hang it over the vertically oriented Weitlaner retractor with a snap on the end of the silk to occlude the vessel. On occasion, accessory ECA branches such as the ascending pharyngeal may be identified on the angiogram and these also need to be isolated with a separate encircling silk suture. It is crucial that all potential sources of backbleeding be identified and controlled before opening the carotid artery since even minor backbleeding will obscure the lumen enough to make shunt placement significantly more difficult.

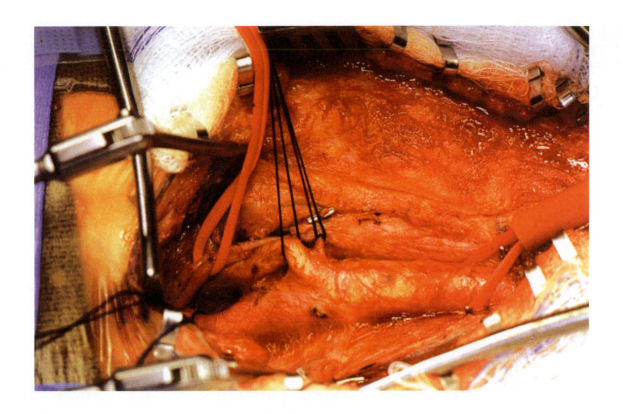

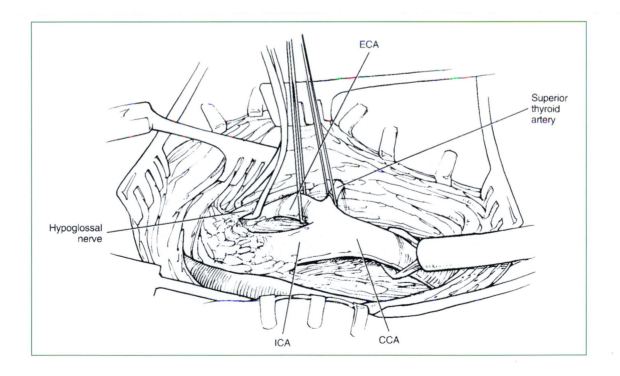

3-28

Isolation of Superior Thyroid Artery—Left Carotid Exposure

A different, closer view shows a superior thyroid artery encircled with Potts tie. In this case, the vessel has already been opened, exposing the plaque and lumen in the common and internal carotid arteries. The isolated hypoglossal nerve is also clearly shown. Note that in this open vessel, no backbleeding can be seen, indicating that Potts tie is effective in securing and obliterating the lumen of the superior thyroid artery.

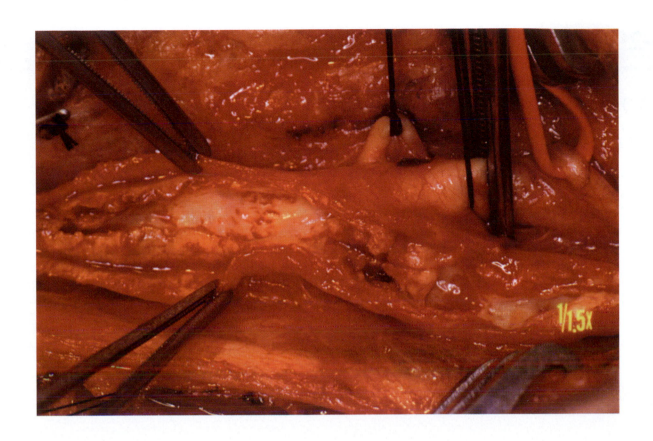

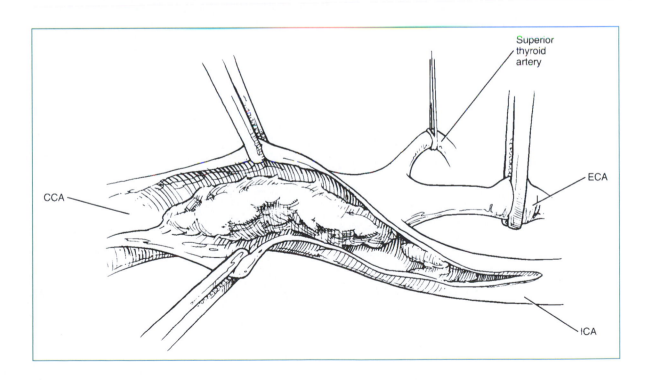

3-29

Isolation of Ascending Pharyngeal Artery (Left)

An ascending pharyngeal artery occasionally arises from the carotid bifurcation rather than from the sidewall of the ECA, and will need to be isolated with a separate 2-0 silk Pott's tie or a bulldog clamp. This figure illustrates one such case. Because this artery was large and was identified on the preoperative arteriograms, I was alerted in advance. The inability to recognize arteries of this type leads to significant back-bleeding when the vessel is opened, obscuring the surgical field and rendering the meticulous dissection necessary for shunt placement and successful endarterectomy more difficult. It is essential to study the arteriogram to identify extra vessels and prevent this sort of complication.

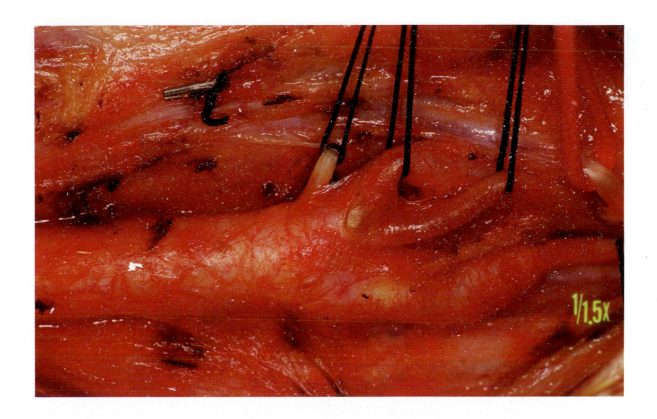

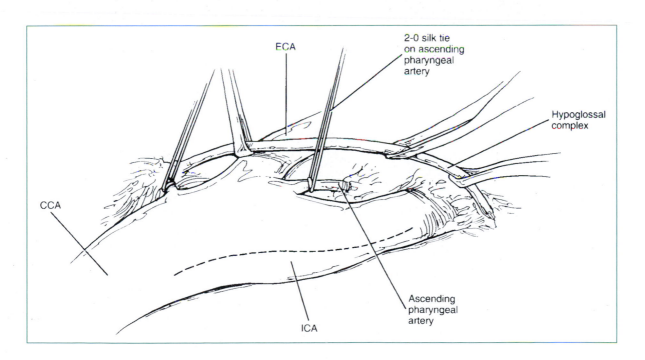

3-30

Isolation of Ascending Pharyngeal Artery (Right)

In this particular case, the figure illustrates another ascending pharyngeal artery that arose from the carotid bifurcation. In this instance, I thought I had isolated all branches of the carotid tree but was troubled by brisk and persistent backbleeding after opening of the carotid system. Because of my inability to complete the repair under these circumstances, I performed an extensive search for the cause of this backbleeding artery, which finally proved to be an ascending pharyngeal artery that was plastered up against the ICA. When this was dissected free, it was possible to place a small bulldog clamp across it, which totally stopped the bleeding.

Note that because of the substitution of a better photograph for this second edition, the artwork depicts an open ICA and a bulldog clamp on the ascending pharyngeal, while the new photograph shows a closed ICA pre-arteriotomy and an encircling silk tie. The principles remain the same.

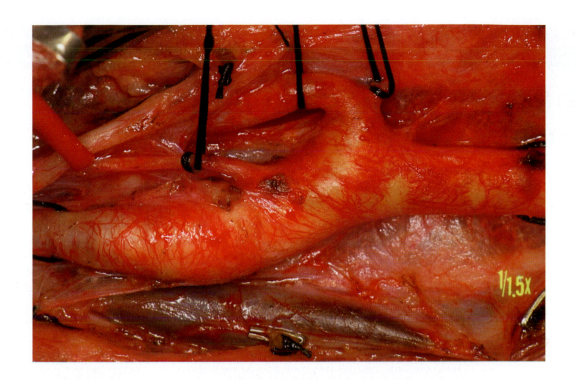

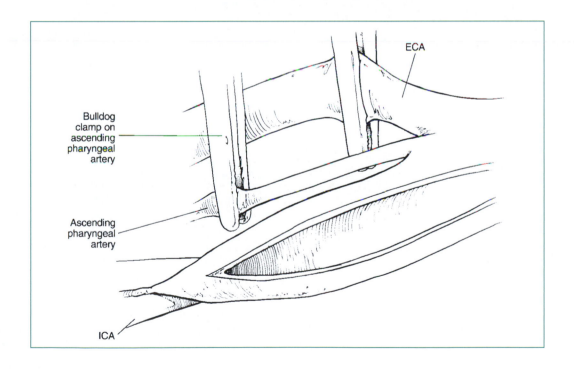

3-31

Tactile and Visual End of Plaque—Left Carotid Exposure

With some experience, it is possible to ascertain the end of the ICA atherosclerotic plaque by visual inspection and tactile palpation of the vessel. It is important to determine this parameter because distal control must be obtained well beyond the end of the plaque in case placement of a shunt is necessary and also because it would be unwise to potentially cross-clamp an ICA across an area of atheroma.

This figure demonstrates the visual cues that indicate the end of the plaque—-in particular, the yellowish shade of the atherosclerotic carotid wall, which turns to a pink/blue color beyond the end of the atheroma. In this case, vascular pickups were placed for demonstration purposes at the portion of the vessel where this transition zone occurs. Likewise, palpation of this vessel would reveal a hard stony plaque in the region of the atheroma and a soft, smooth pliable vessel distal to it. Note that the silk tie encircling the ICA has been placed well above the end of the plaque and a nice high ICA exposure has been achieved. In this particular figure, the vagus nerve lying lateral and deep to the ICA can also be seen.

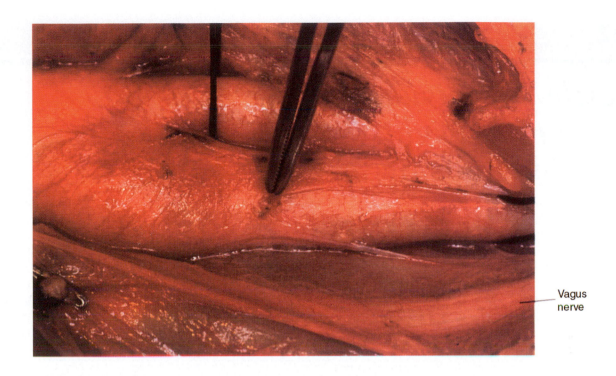

Vagus nerve

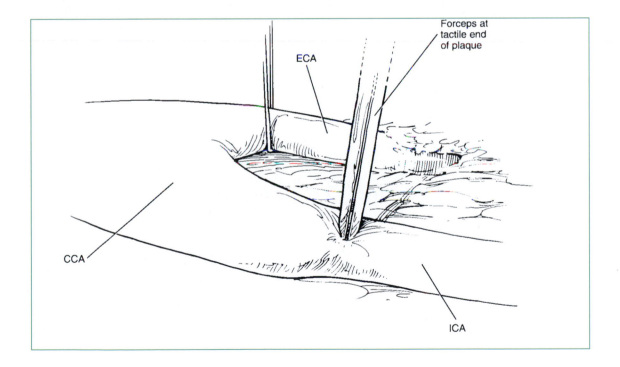

Forceps at tactile end of plaque

ECA

CCA

ICA

3-32

Tactile and Visual End of Plaque—Right Carotid Exposure

A low-power, more general view of a right carotid artery ready for cross-clamping provides a good example of the visual end of atheromatous plaque. The bayonet illustrates the end of the tactile and visual atheroma, and an ICA exposure was developed well above this region.

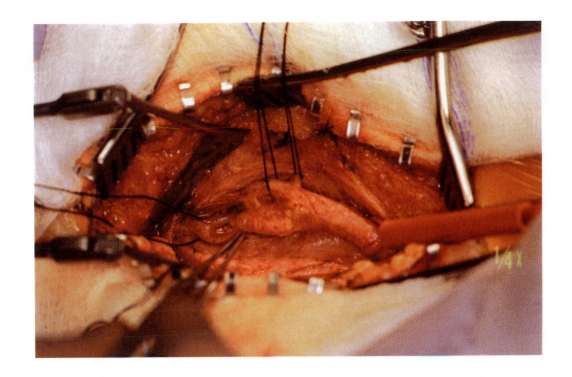

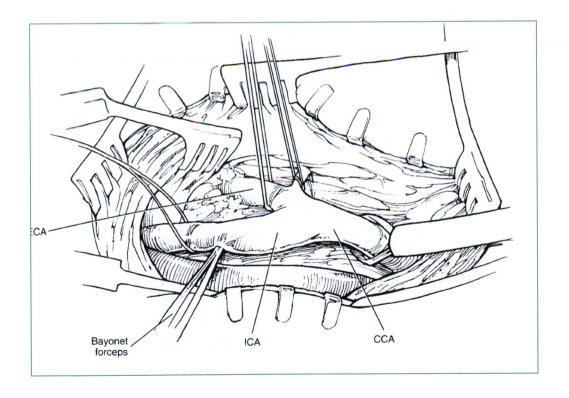

3-33

Extensive Plaque Erosion into the Adventitial Layer

We occasionally encounter atheromatous plaques so extensive and erosive that they create an outpouching type ulceration into the outer layers of the carotid. Depending on surgeon preference, a number of strategies can be called upon to fix this. In this particular case, which is one of my earlier ones, I excised this area of outpouching and did an end-to-end anastomosis of the wall with interrupted 6-0 Prolene sutures. Today, I think instead I would simply excise the wall widely and use the Hemashield patch to reconstruct a widely patent lumen. Without one of these strategies, the residual wall after endarterectomy would have been sufficiently thin that I think the patient would have been at risk for blowout if managed with only simple conventional endarterectomy and primary repair. The surgeon must be prepared to embrace unusual and creative strategies when faced with these types of variants.

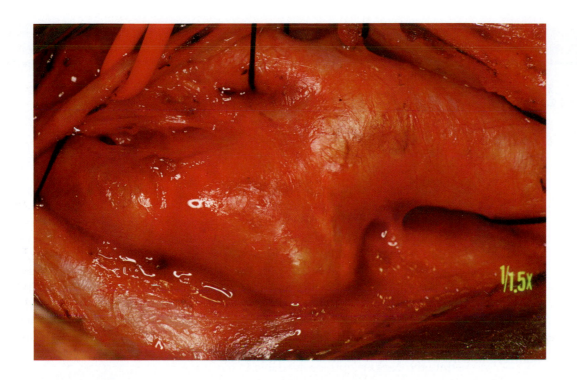

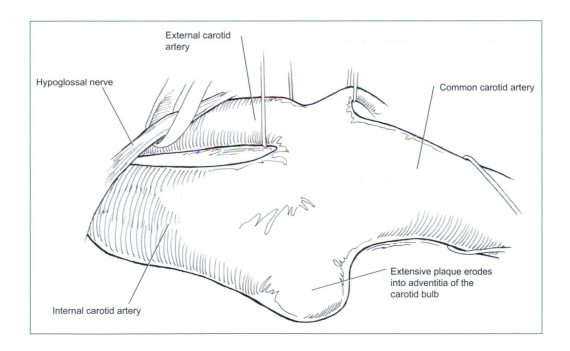

3-34

Javid Clamp Around Internal Carotid Artery

One method of securing a shunt in place is with a small Javid clamp. When the high exposure of the ICA is obtained and the silk suture is passed around it for control, it is important to ascertain that adequate space has been left for placement of the Javid clamp to secure an indwelling shunt if necessary. As shown here, a small Javid clamp is placed from the lateral side and encircles the vessel as a test. The clamp can then be closed around the vessel, securing the plastic shunt tubing in place. Without this type of preparation, it is possible that a filmy veil of carotid sheath tissue behind the carotid artery will interfere with and prevent successful placement of the Javid clamp later on and the resultant backbleeding around the shunt will be particularly troublesome.

I previously used Javid clamps but have switched to my own clamp design now (see Figs. 3-35 and 3-50). The Javid clamp illustrations are retained, however, to demonstrate the various options available to the surgeon.

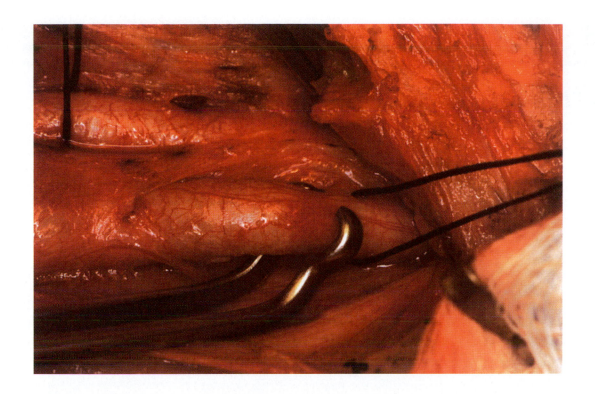

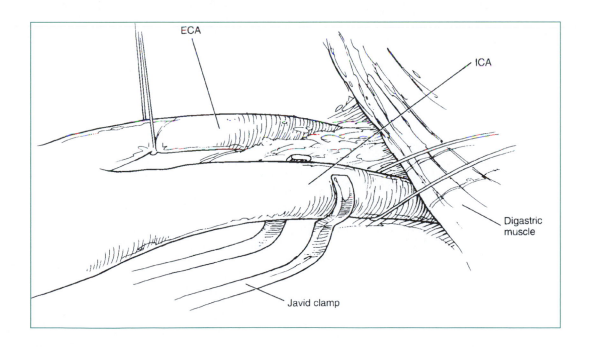

ECA

ICA

Digastric
muscle

Javid clamp

3-35

Loftus Shunt Clamps

This illustration shows three models of a spring loaded internal carotid shunt clamp of the author's design, manufactured by Scanlan Instruments of St. Paul, MN. I previously used a Javid type clamp to secure the ICA around an indwelling shunt, but I was unhappy with the long handle protruding into the carotid bed. These simple clamps pinch down gently and encircle the ICA, preventing backbleeding from the distal vessel. They closing force is gentle to prevent intimal damage, and they come in various angles (as illustrated here) to allow them to be custom sized and to remain unobtrusive in the wound.

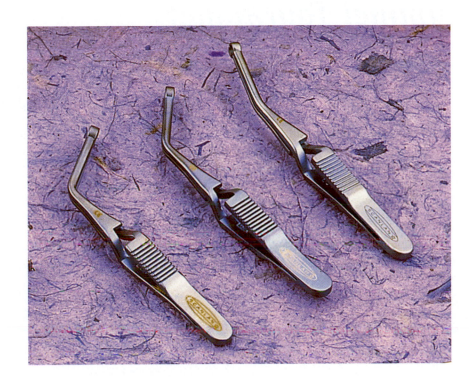

3-36

Placement of Cross-Clamp Below Rummel Tourniquet

My technique of shunt insertion will be described later. This drawing is intended to illustrate that in preparation for placement of a shunt it is essential that the Rummel tourniquet that will secure the shunt in place be at least 1 cm (hopefully farther) distal to the DeBakey cross-clamp. This entails dissection of a fair amount of CCA to obtain a good proximal location for placement of the cross clamp. The reason for this is that in order to avoid copious bleeding with placement of the shunt in the CCA, it is my preference to place the shunt down in the lumen of the vessel through the Rummel tourniquet loop until it abuts against the cross-clamp. The loop can then be securely snugged down around it before the cross-clamp is removed. When the cross-clamp is then removed, there is essentially no bleeding because the shunt has already been secured, but it is still possible to slide the shunt farther down the CCA as it slips quite nicely through the loop. In this way I have converted a procedure that formerly produced copious bleeding into an essentially bloodless task.

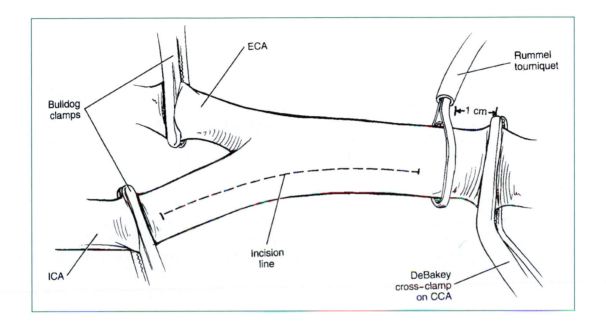

3-37

Incision Along Common and Internal Carotid Arteries (Blue Line)—Left Carotid Exposure

Shown is a carotid artery fully prepared for cross-clamping. Note that the superior thyroid artery and the external, internal, and common carotid arteries have all been secured with their respective loops and silk ties. Adequate exposure of the distal ICA has been obtained, and a long segment of CCA is available proximal to the vessel loop so that the DeBakey clamp may be well below the vessel loop in case a shunt is needed.

Using a sterile marking pen, I draw a line indicating the area of proposed incision in the carotid artery to prevent a jagged suture line if the vessel rotates as it is opened and to facilitate the repair.

After the encephalographer is notified of impending cross-clamping, I prefer to use a bulldog clamp to close the ICA first, followed immediately by DeBakey cross-clamping of the CCA and a second bulldog clamp applied to the ECA below the level of any branches except the superior thyroid artery. Closing the ICA first prevents any plaque that might become dislodged by the CCA cross-clamp from entering the cranial circulation.

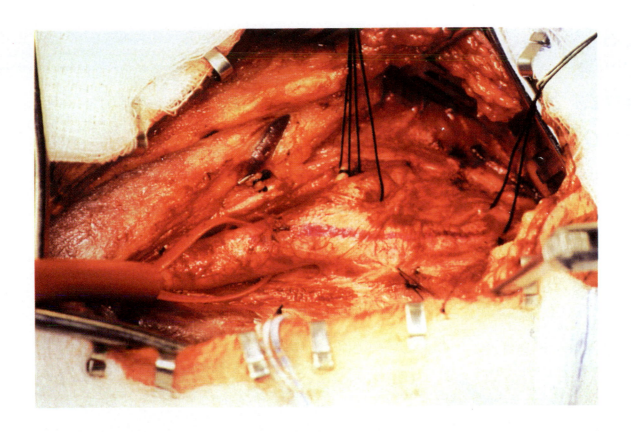

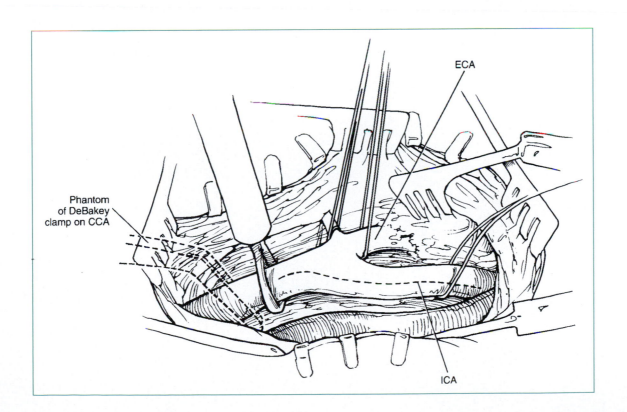

3-38

Potts Scissors Opening—Left Carotid Exposure

After cross-clamping, a stab incision is made in the proximal CCA with a No. 11 knife. Suction is used to evacuate all blood from the vessel, and backbleeding should be non-existent. The lumen can then be visualized, and the lower blade of a Potts scissors is introduced to cut a straight line up along the previously drawn blue line into the ICA.

When the plaque is thick, it is possible to get into a false plane and it becomes critical to ascertain that the lower blade of Potts scissors is within the vessel lumen at all times. In cases in which this is difficult, the ICA bulldog clamp can be briefly released, allowing some backbleeding and demonstrating the ICA lumen.

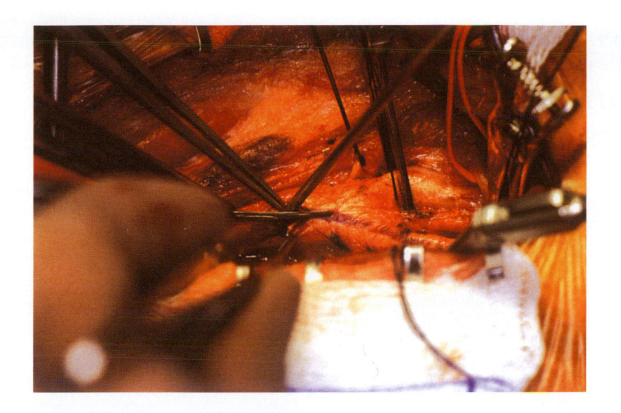

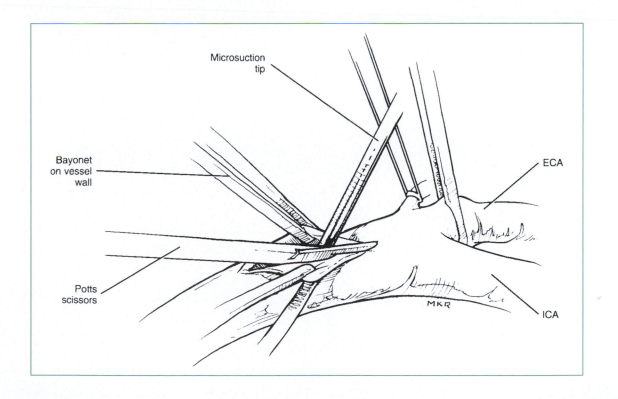

Microsuction tip

Bayonet on vessel wall

Potts scissors

ECA

ICA

MKR

3-39

Potts Scissors Opening Vessel—Left Carotid Exposure

A somewhat lower-powered view again demonstrates the Potts scissors having entered the carotid bulb and coming up the ICA along the midline of the vessel. It is important to avoid any deviation from the midline in the region of the carotid bulb when using the Potts scissors and instead to go directly up the center, since an incision closer to the crotch of the carotid bulb will render the repair more difficult to achieve in hemostatic fashion.

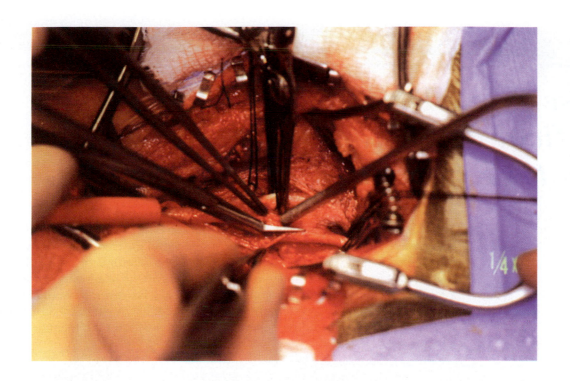

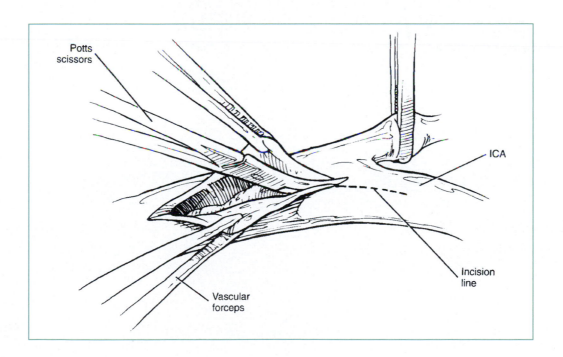

3-40

False Plane Demonstrated with Penfield Retractor—Right Carotid Exposure

This figure is an example of a false plane that can develop in the process of opening the ICA lumen. The Penfield No. 4 retractor is situated in the true lumen of the vessel, and it can be seen that the Potts scissors went through the atheroma of a false plane and eventually burst into the true lumen in the ICA. There are no untoward consequences from a false dissection of this type in opening the vessel; however, it should be emphasized that the surgeon must ascertain the true lumen of the ICA either by direct inspection or visualization of backbleeding before any attempt at shunt placement.

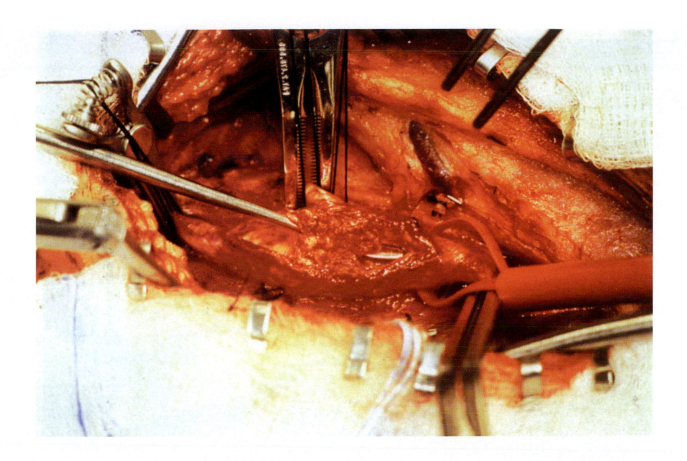

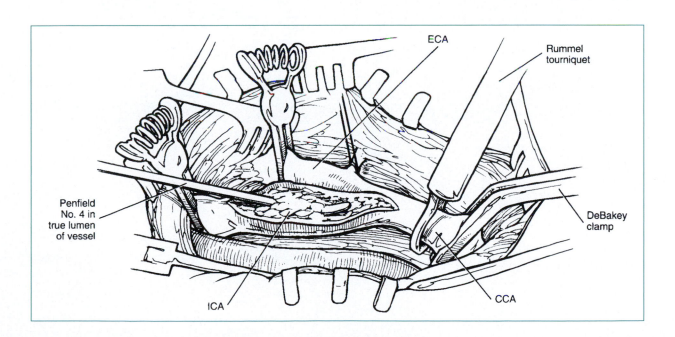

ECA

Rummel
tourniquet

Penfield
No. 4 in
true lumen
of vessel

DeBakey
clamp

ICA

CCA

3-41

Focal Plaque in Proximal Internal Carotid Artery—Left Carotid Exposure

A focal tight stenosis at the carotid bulb is shown. There is no extensive plaque either down the CCA or up the ICA, making this a relatively simple and straightforward exposure and plaque removal. However, the brown, discolored area of carotid plaque indicates the presence of intraplaque hemorrhage and an active plaque that no doubt was responsible for the patient's symptoms. This is type of soft, friable plaque that is so often associated with intraplaque hemorrhage.

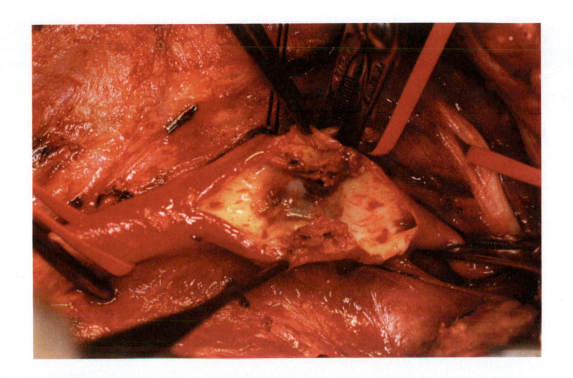

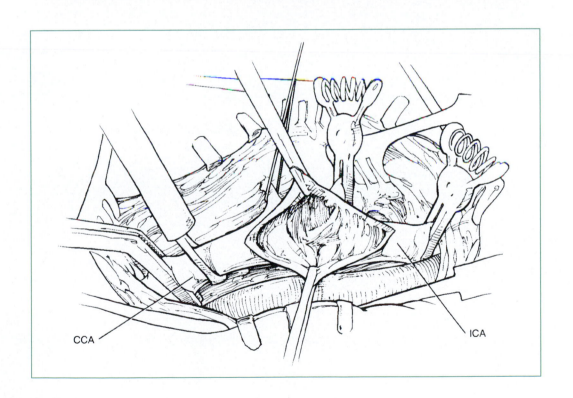

CCA   ICA

3-42

Long, Extensive Common Carotid Artery/Internal Carotid Artery Plaque

Shown is a long atherosclerotic plaque that extends far down the CCA and also a good distance up the ICA. The repair involved a time-consuming, extensive arteriotomy; otherwise the operation was straightforward. I thought it was important in this case to take the CCA arteriotomy low enough for all ulcerated areas of the plaque to be removed.

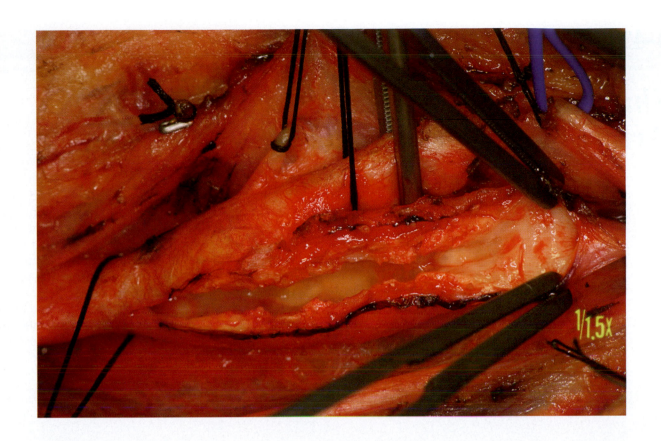

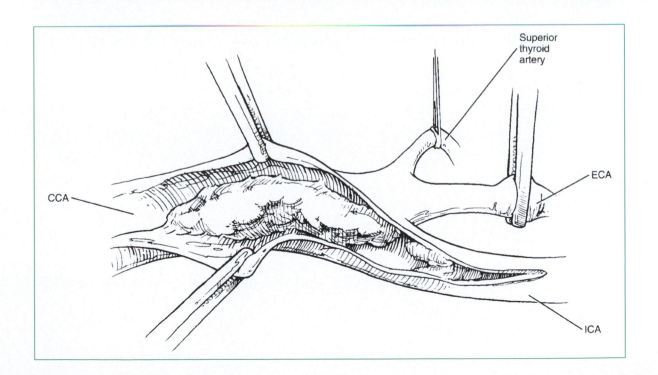

3-43

Shunt in Common Carotid Artery/Internal Carotid Artery

I previously used a shunt fashioned from a pediatric No. 8 feeding tube cut 15 cm in length. As we have said, this style shunt is now manufactured as a "Loftus shunt" (see Fig. 3-50). A preexisting black dot at the middle of the tube becomes the midpoint of the shunt after it is placed. The dot serves as a marker for positioning in the center of the lumen to prevent unnoticed cephalad migration. I find this less cumbersome than placing a string around the shunt, which may interfere with the repair. The shunt is secured by a Rummel tourniquet in the CCA (Fig. 3-36) and by a small Javid clamp or the Loftus pinch clamp in the distal ICA, as previously described (Figs. 3-34 and 3-35). The hand-held Doppler probe can be applied to this exposed shunt tubing, and an audible flow signal will be faintly heard, confirming shunt patency. Shunt function is also assessed by noting return of monitoring parameters to baseline (whether EEG, TCD, SSEP, or other methods are used).

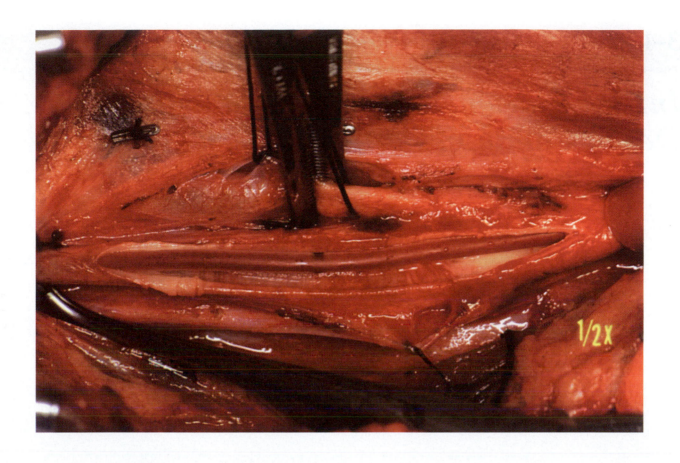

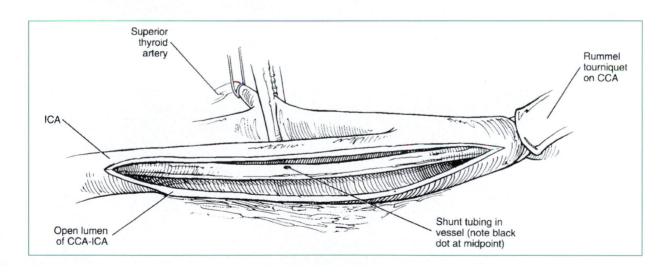

3-44

Initial Placement of Shunt Down Common Carotid Artery

As mentioned earlier in the text, it is my preference to place a shunt in the CCA first. I have ensured that the cross-clamp is at least 1 cm below the Rummel tourniquet. This drawing illustrates placement of the shunt down the CCA and through the Rummel tourniquet until it abuts against the clamp. The Rummel tourniquet is then secured as shown in the drawing, after which the clamp can be released and the shunt can be advanced farther caudally until essentially all of the shunt is down the CCA.

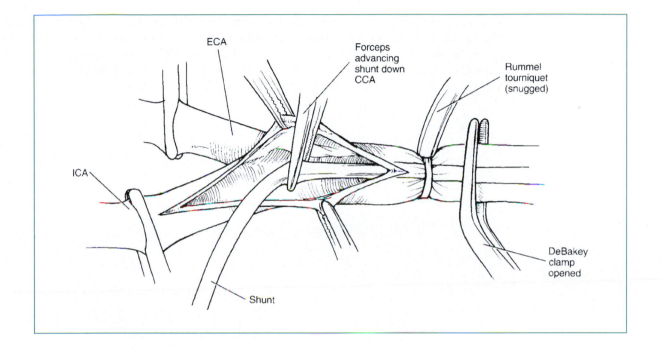

3-45

Securing of Shunt in Common Carotid Artery

This is a detailed view of the securing of the shunt in the CCA. When the shunt is placed, the DeBakey clamp is not removed from the CCA, but rather the shunt is placed down to the level of the DeBakey clamp and then the Rummel tourniquet is secured around it. After this, the DeBakey clamp can be removed without significant bleeding, and the shunt is advanced in retrograde fashion down the CCA.

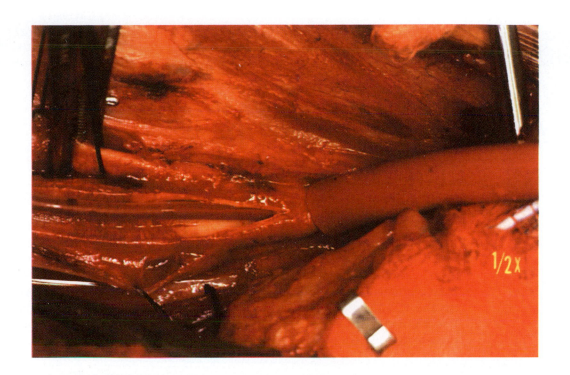

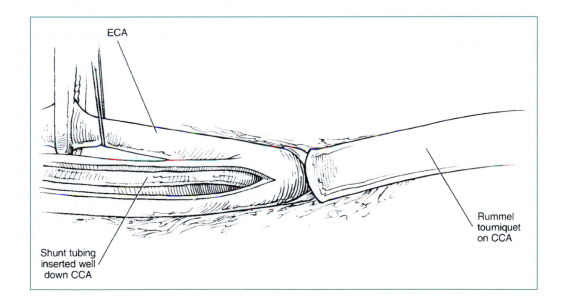

ECA

Shunt tubing
inserted well
down CCA

Rummel
tourniquet
on CCA

3-46

Bleeding and Evacuation of Shunt Before Placement in Internal Carotid Artery

Once the shunt has been placed and secured in the CCA and has slid down satisfactorily, the DeBakey forceps that are holding the plastic tubing closed are released until the entire shunt lumen is filled with a solid column of blood and all air and debris have been evacuated from it. In this fashion, one can be certain that no atheroma dislodged from placement of the shunt remains in the lumen where it might inadvertently be sent up the ICA. The ability to evacuate any possible atheroma is the reason I place this shunt in the CCA first, and only when I am certain that there is no foreign material present do I place it in the ICA.

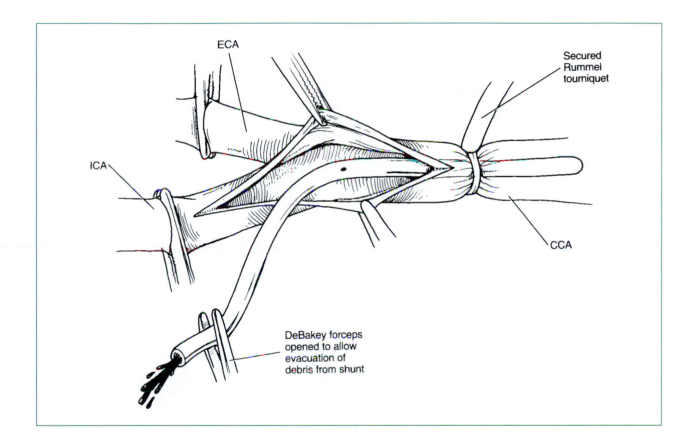

3-47

Placement of Shunt in Distal Internal Carotid Artery

When the shunt lumen has been evacuated, suction is used to completely empty the ICA of blood or residual debris. The assistant then removes the bulldog clamp allowing the ICA to backbleed. At the same time, the shunt is advanced up the backbleeding ICA in the gentlest possible fashion; when it has been initially placed, the DeBakey forceps can be removed allowing the shunt to bleed forward as well. This process of antegrade bleeding in the shunt blows open the ICA to some extent and prevents the shunt from abutting against the vessel wall. If there is the least bit of resistance to passage of the shunt, I stop, remove it, and try again, but it usually slides up quite freely without a problem. The shunt is advanced until the black dot appears in the center of the wound at the region of the carotid bulb. This black dot has $7\frac{1}{2}$ cm of shunt on either side of it and ensures that the shunt is properly placed. It serves as a marker throughout the operative procedure to prevent unnoticed cephalad migration of the shunt with possible dislodgment from the CCA.

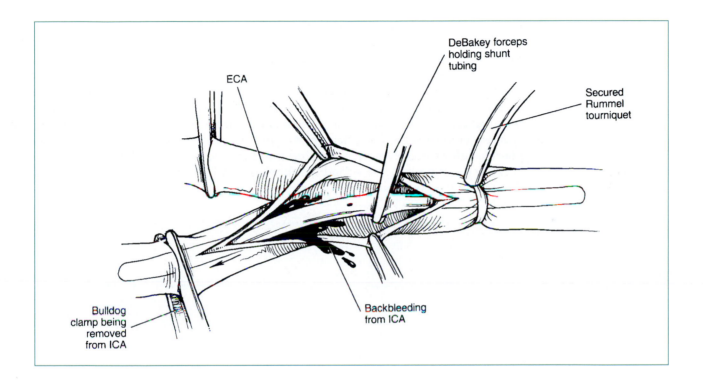

ECA

DeBakey forceps
holding shunt
tubing

Secured
Rummel
tourniquet

Bulldog
clamp being
removed
from ICA

Backbleeding
from ICA

3-48

Potential for Intimal Damage from Placement of Shunt

I have emphasized that the shunt needs to be inserted with the gentlest of techniques in the ICA. As described previously, I never force a shunt if it does not slide readily up in the ICA because the advancing end of the shunt may theoretically roughen or damage the intimal high in the ICA beyond the area of the arteriotomy, leading to dissection of the ICA with consequent thrombosis and embolic phenomena and devastating neurologic consequences for the patient. This potential damage is illustrated in this drawing in which forceful insertion of the shunt is shown to raise an intimal flap. Of course, this is an extremely uncommon phenomenon. In the vast majority of my cases, the shunt is placed with absolutely no difficulty up into the ICA so long as the ICA is allowed to backbleed during the process and the shunt is held open so that antegrade flow blows the vessel walls apart and out of harm's way.

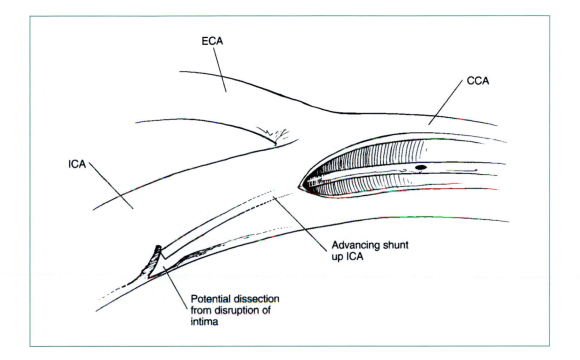

3-49

Securing of Shunt in Internal Carotid Artery

When the shunt has been successfully placed in the ICA, it can be secured with a small Javid clamp or with a Loftus pinch clamp to prevent backbleeding around it. This clamp has been previously sized in the wound as shown in Figs. 3-34 and 3-35.

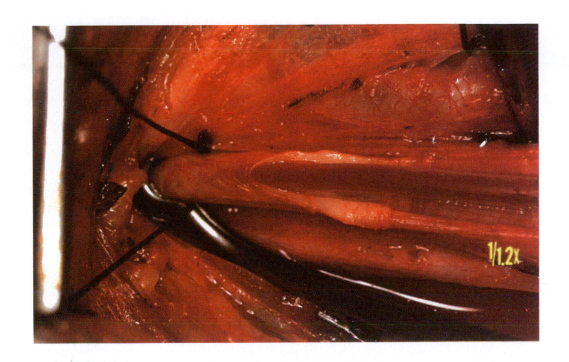

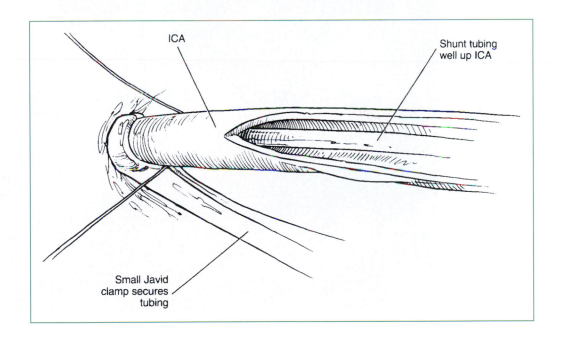

ICA

Shunt tubing
well up ICA

Small Javid
clamp secures
tubing

3-50

Loftus Type Carotid Shunt in Place—Two Views

The Loftus type shunt (Integra Neuroscience, Plainsboro, NJ) is a straight silastic tube chamfered at the ICA end for easy placement, and with a built-up bulb at the CCA end to anchor it in the Rummel tourniquet. There is a black line at the center of the shunt to indicate migration during the case. In these two photos we illustrate the shunt in place with the black line properly placed at the center of the arteriotomy. We also show the shunt being secured by the Loftus type pinch clamps (Fig. 3-35) in the ICA: in (B), at the right edge of the frame, the shunt can be seen to be secured in the CCA by the 0 silk tie within the Rummel tourniquet.

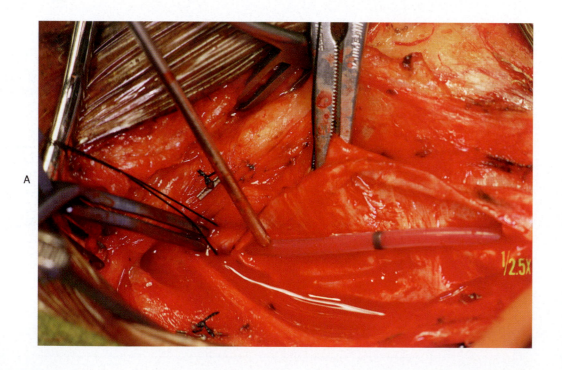

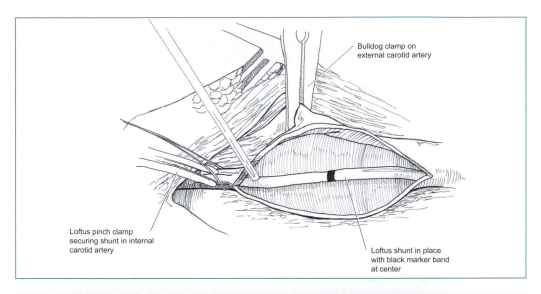

Bulldog clamp on external carotid artery

Loftus pinch clamp securing shunt in internal carotid artery

Loftus shunt in place with black marker band at center

B

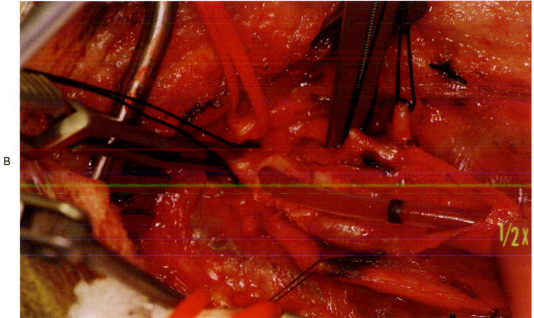

Bulldog clamp on external carotid artery

Hypoglossal nerve

Superior thyroid artery

Loftus type shunt in place with marker band in center of arteriotomy

Loftus pinch clamp securing shunt in internal carotid artery

Rummel tourniquet on common carotid artery

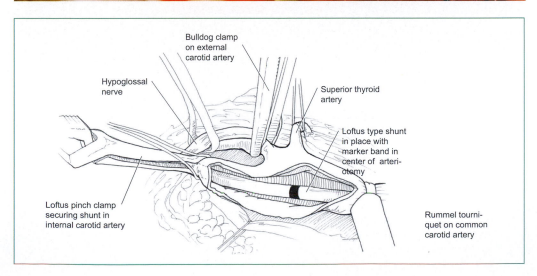

3-51

Evaluation of Shunt Function

There are a number of ways to evaluate shunt function and ensure that antegrade flow is present. The simplest is application of a hand-held Doppler probe to the shunt tubing. The audible flow signal, although faint, has confirmed patency in every case in my experience. Shunt function can also be ascertained by various monitoring techniques, and I anticipate that the EEG or similar monitoring technique will return to baseline after satisfactory placement of an indwelling shunt. TCD velocities are also expected to improve to at least 50% or more of their baseline values with proper placement of a shunt.

If monitoring parameters do not improve once a shunt has been placed, a careful assessment of possible shunt malfunction, whether through thrombosis or abutment against the distal ICA wall, is needed.

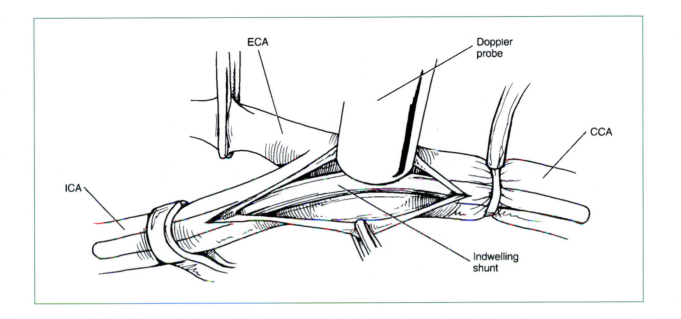

3-52

Repair with Shunt in Place

In this case, the ICA repair is nearly complete and only the CCA and bulb portions of the shunt are visible. Note that the black dot continues to mark the midpoint of the arteriotomy. In this procedure, the Rummel tourniquet did not prove adequate to secure the shunt without some degree of minor, but annoying, antegrade bleeding, and a large Javid clamp was placed around the CCA as a backup. This was an unusual occurrence since the vessel loop or 0 silk encased in the Rummel tourniquet typically stops bleeding around the shunt.

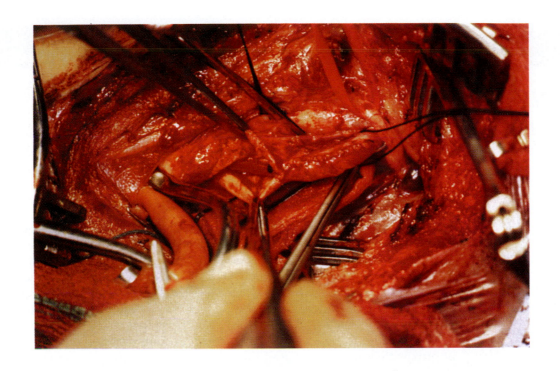

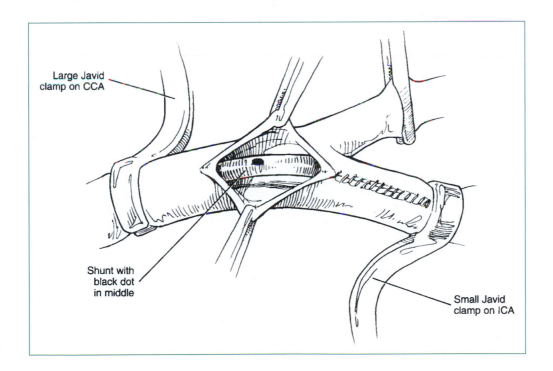

Large Javid
clamp on CCA

Shunt with
black dot
in middle

Small Javid
clamp on ICA

3-53

Plaque Removal Begins at Lateral Edge—Left Carotid Exposure

When the arteriotomy is complete and the decision has been made whether or not to shunt, plaque removal begins. I start at the lateral edge of the vessel using a Penfield No. 4 microdissector or a Freer dissector and rub gently back and forth along the vessel wall. In a primary case, it usually falls into a cleavage plane just outside the atheromatous intimal plaque, which is easily dissected. Gentle dissection is required to avoid buttonholing the residual vessel wall, which may be quite thin. I prefer the Penfield microdissector, which is always turned medially so that no sharp edge extends through the plaque into the vessel wall. The dissection continues in a circumferential fashion approximately halfway around the vessel, and the same process is repeated on the medial side. Dissection also proceeds in a rostral-caudal direction in an attempt to gently free up both the ICA attachments of the plaque and the CCA, which is prepared for sharp transection.

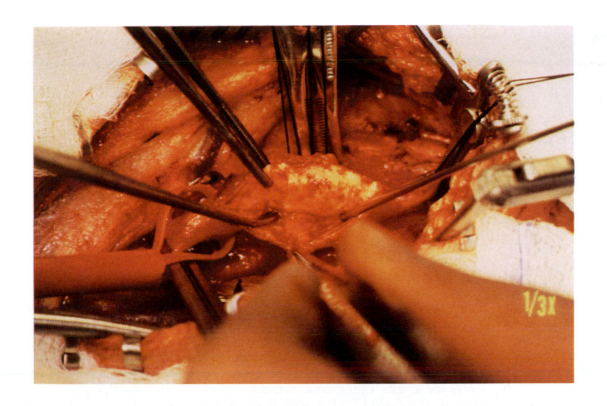

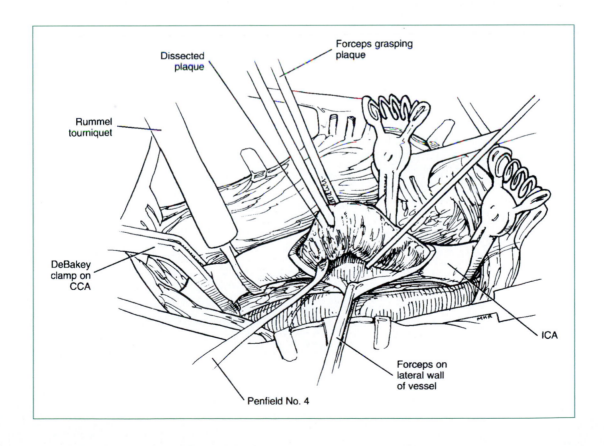

3-54

Sharp Transection in Common Carotid Artery—Right Carotid Exposure

When the plaque has been dissected circumferentially from the lumen of the carotid bulb and CCA, it is usually not possible to follow it far enough down the CCA to obtain a feathered edge, as is done in the ICA. I prefer to sharply transect the CCA plaque at the point where the caudad dissection ends. This can be accomplished with either a No. 15 blade or, as in this case, Church scissors. Once again, it is important to identify the back wall of the vessel so that it is not inadvertently buttonholed by either cutting technique. Once the plaque has been sharply removed from the CCA, it can be held up with the vascular forceps and removed from the internal and external carotid arteries.

It should also be kept in mind that complete plaque removal is difficult if the incision abuts against the DeBakey clamp. For this reason, as well as for avoiding difficulty with the repairs, I am always certain that the CCA cross-clamp (or Rummel tourniquet if a shunt is used) is well proximal (at least 1 to 2 cm) to the end of the arteriotomy.

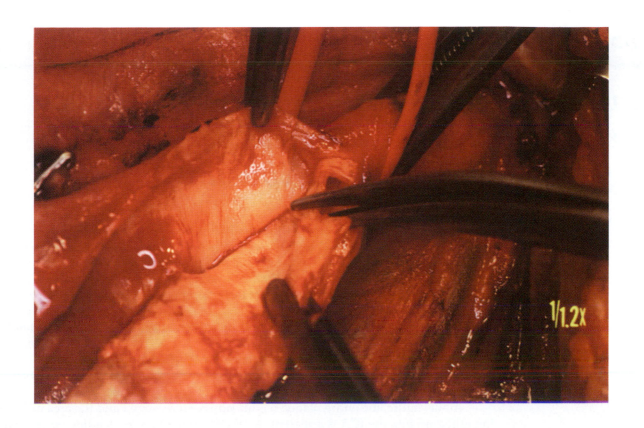

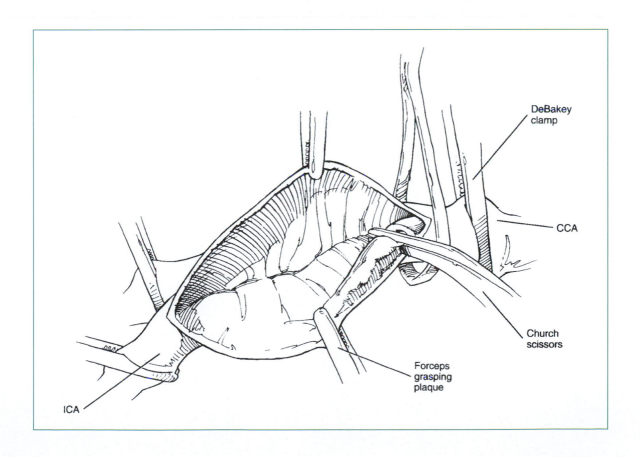

3-55

Plaque Removal from Internal Carotid Artery (Feathered Edge)—Right Carotid Exposure

The technique of plaque removal from the ICA differs somewhat from the technique used in the CCA. Whereas sharp transection is nearly always needed to remove the proximal CCA plaque, in the ICA the plaque often feathers out quite nicely during dissection, leaving a smooth edge of intima up into the unexposed area of the ICA. Also, unlike the CCA, it is important to dissect the atheromatous plaque to its full extent so that no residual atheroma is left behind.

In my experience there is often a "tail" of thickened yellow intima that extends up the posterior wall of the ICA, and it is this "tail" that needs to be carefully feathered free. In some cases, the tail will extend above the level of the arteriotomy. If there is a possibility of inadequate feathering, the arteriotomy must be extended for inspection of the wall.

In this figure, the entire plaque has already been removed and the area of feathering going up into the ICA is apparent. A "shelf" with a tattered leading edge needs to be cleaned up and tacked down with 6-0 Prolene double-armed tacking sutures. I believe it is important that shelves such as this be tacked to prevent the possibility of dissection by the antegrade column of blood flow when clamps are removed. Also visible in this figure are several small fragments that will need to be removed in circumferential fashion before closing the arteriotomy. This is a good example of recommended technique, with the arteriotomy taken well above the plaque into a normal area of the ICA.

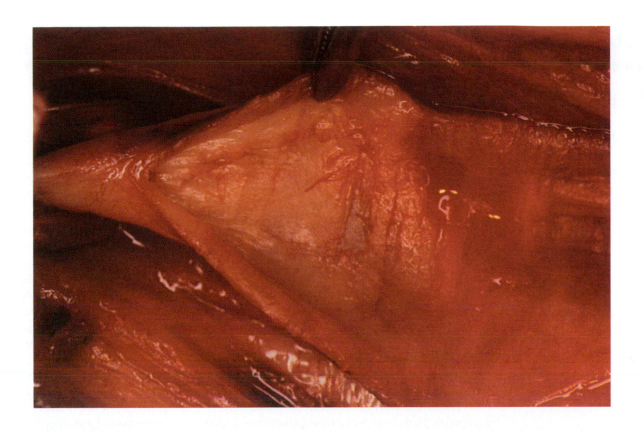

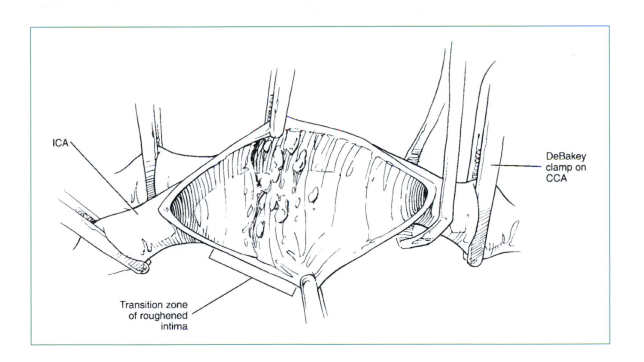

ICA

DeBakey
clamp on
CCA

Transition zone
of roughened
intima

3-56

Plaque Removal from External Carotid Artery—Left Carotid Exposure

In the majority of CEA procedures, the plaque can be removed from the ECA without having to open that vessel as a separate incision. Once the plaque is freed from the common and internal carotid arteries, the remaining plaque wall is grasped with vascular forceps to pull down the plaque from the ECA orifice. This basically inverts the ECA lumen as the plaque is pulled back and usually results in a clean distal break-off up in the region of the occluding bulldog clamp. If the plaque does not immediately release, the bulldog clamp can be temporarily opened, allowing the plaque to be popped down from the distal ECA. It is also helpful to sweep around the interface between the plaque and ECA residual vessel wall with either a Penfield No. 4 dissector or a curved mosquito clamp, thereby freeing up some of these atherosclerotic fragments. It is necessary to open the ECA separately only if the plaque does not come out easily in this fashion.

When the plaque has been removed, it is important to check for remaining loose fragments, both under direct visualization and tactilely, by passing a curved mosquito clamp up into the now denuded area of the ECA. Any fragments can then be pulled off in circumferential fashion.

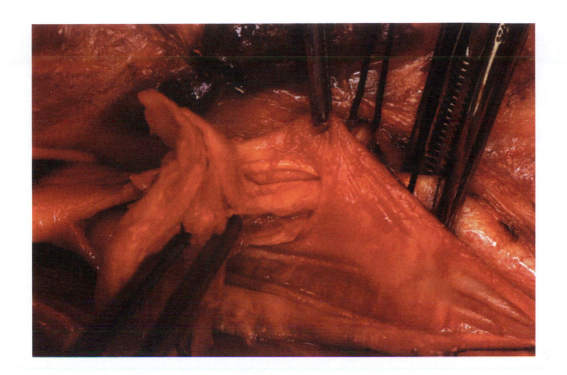

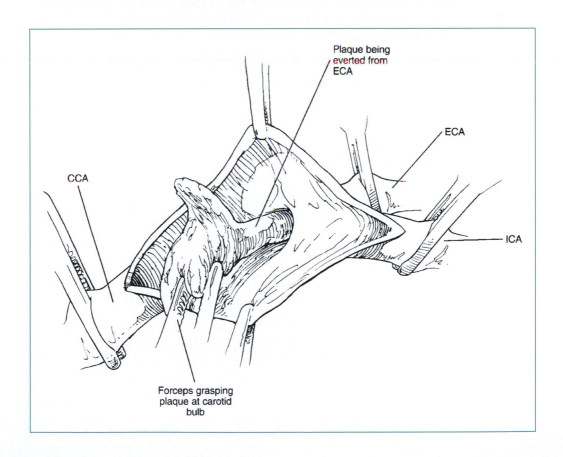

Plaque being
everted from
ECA

ECA

CCA

ICA

Forceps grasping
plaque at carotid
bulb

3-57

Opening of External Carotid Artery—Inadequate Feathering

Marsupialization of the plaque from the ECA is usually sufficient to ensure a clean break-off. However, if fragments can be palpated or a rough edge can be demonstrated on inspection of the endarterectomized ECA with a curved clamp, I do not hesitate to open the ECA with a separate arteriotomy that begins at the carotid bifurcation, extends straight up the ECA, and is performed in the same fashion as the ICA arteriotomy, creating a Y-shaped arteriotomy defect that needs to be closed in that manner. Inattention to detail in the performance of the ECA endarterectomy can be the source of thrombus formation and later embolization up the ICA, or it may lead to a dissection of the ECA (illustrated in Fig. 2-21), which may ultimately cause thrombosis of the entire carotid tree with devastating consequences for the patient.

In the case illustrated here, the ECA has been opened as a separate limb of the original arteriotomy. The Penfield No. 4 dissector reveals a tail of plaque, which was incompletely removed in the marsupialization technique and which now must be dissected free, well up the ECA to the level of the bulldog clamp in just the same fashion as for the ICA endarterectomy. Likewise, if plaque appears to extend beyond the bulldog clamp, this can be released briefly, allowing the plaque to be pulled back for a clean distal break-off. I cannot emphasize strongly enough the need for attention to detail in the performance of the ECA endarterectomy and would urge that the ECA be opened in every case in which even the slightest concern exists regarding thorough plaque removal.

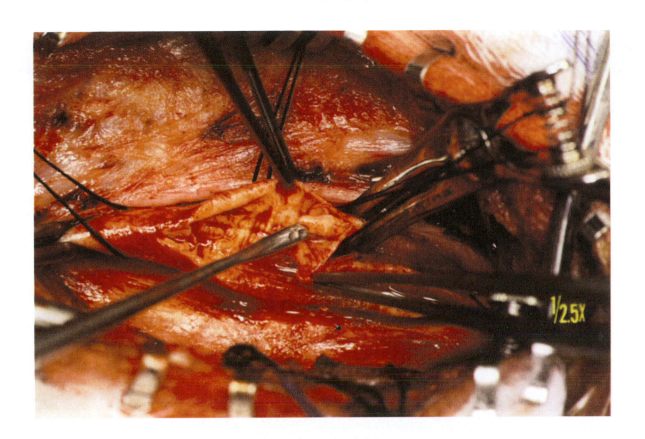

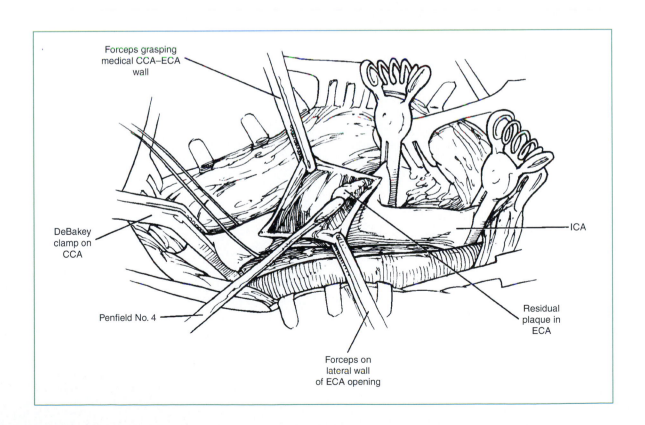

Forceps grasping
medical CCA–ECA
wall

DeBakey
clamp on
CCA

Penfield No. 4

Forceps on
lateral wall
of ECA opening

ICA

Residual
plaque in
ECA

3-58

Opening of External Carotid Artery—Inadequate Feathering

This is another illustration of, in this case, a right CEA in which the ECA was opened as a separate arteriotomy. An area of rough plaque that did not readily marsupialize can be seen right at the orifice of the ECA. I thought a formal endarterectomy was necessary to adequately clean up the ECA and, as shown in this figure, made a separate incision directly up the ECA to the level of the 2-0 silk tie.

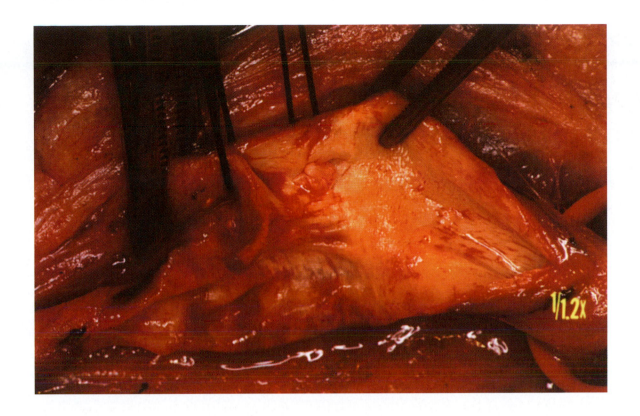

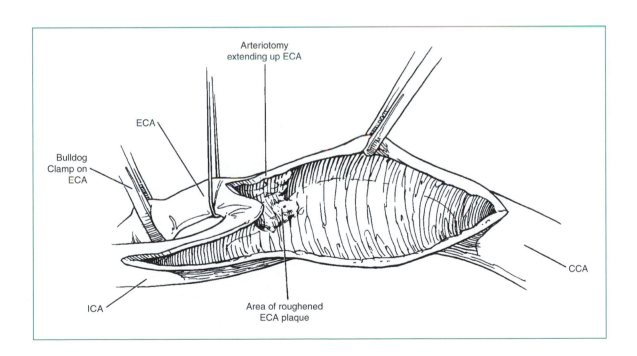

3-59

Opening of External Carotid Artery Because of Poor Doppler Signal

In this case I had completed the internal carotid repair with Hemashield patch grafting. On final auscultation (after declamping), the Doppler signal from the ECA was high-pitched consistent with persistent stenosis. Fortunately a shunt had not been required. The clamps were re-applied and the ECA was opened over a short distal segment and residual plaque was removed. Following this strategy, as previously illustrated, a primary ECA repair without patch graft was performed, although in this case it did not extend back to the carotid bulb.

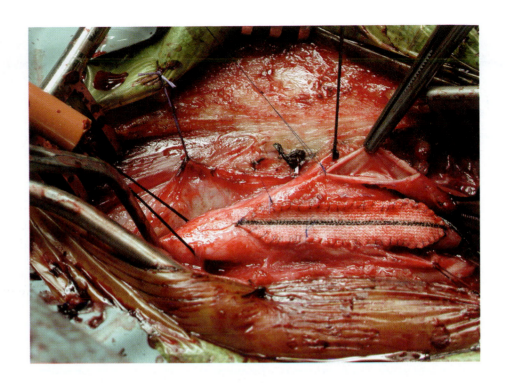

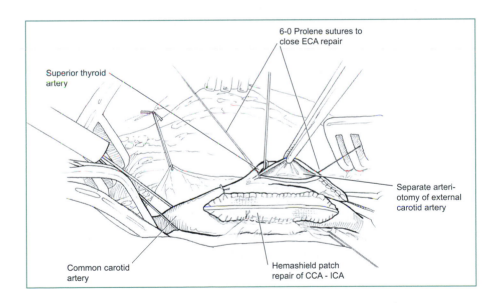

6-0 Prolene sutures to
close ECA repair

Superior thyroid
artery

Separate arteri-
otomy of external
carotid artery

Common carotid
artery

Hemashield patch
repair of CCA - ICA

3-60

Opening of External Carotid Artery—Repair

This is a left CEA in which it was necessary to open and repair the ECA as a separate incision. In this case the common to internal carotid arteriotomy remains open and the denuded area of vascular wall following plaque removal can be seen. A suture line is begun in the ECA and brought down in continuous, nonlocking fashion to the region of the carotid bulb where it is secured to a separately thrown single 6-0 Prolene stitch. The long tail of this stitch is then tied to one of the limbs of the main suture line when the common and internal carotid arteries are repaired. It is important to note that when I do open the ECA separately, I repair it first since there is a rather limited amount of time available for completion of the arterial suture line at the junction of the common and internal arteries, particularly in shunted cases.

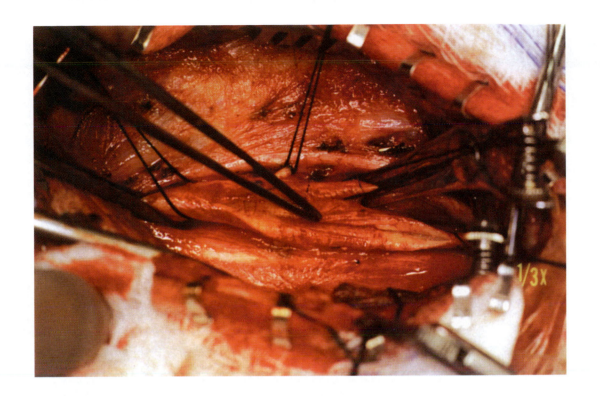

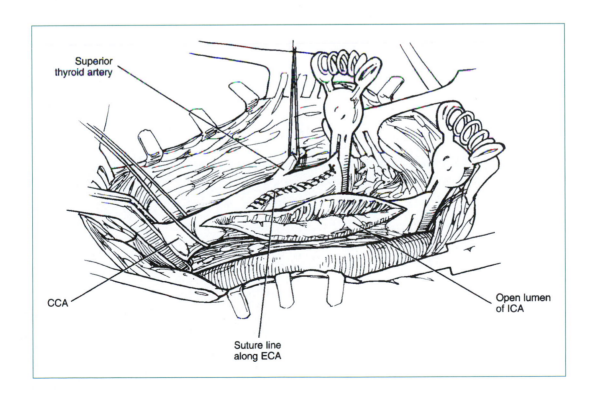

Superior
thyroid artery

Open lumen
of ICA

CCA

Suture line
along ECA

3-61

Completed External Carotid Artery Repair in a Case with Internal Carotid Artery Hemashield Patch

This photograph shows the final result in a case where an ICA Hemashield patch was used and the ECA was opened secondarily for poor Doppler signal. The field is dry and the repair is secure at both the primary and the patch closure sites. The clamps have been removed and flow is re-established with no bleeding or leaks.

This photograph also illustrates well the use of the 4 retention sutures to hold open the carotid sheath and improve the vascular exposure.

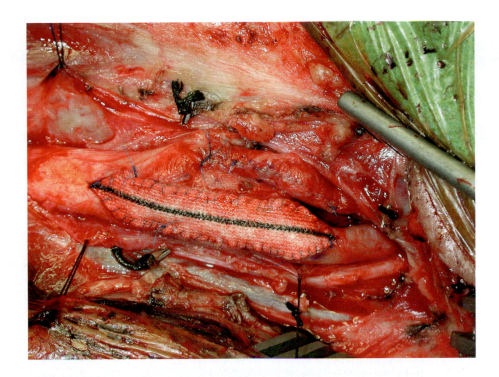

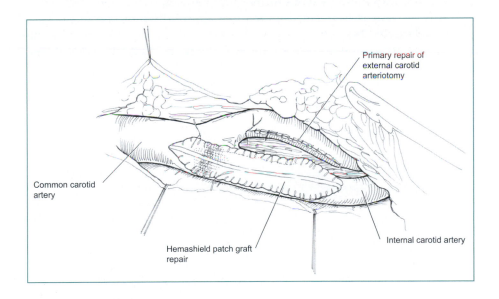

Primary repair of external carotid arteriotomy

Common carotid artery

Hemashield patch graft repair

Internal carotid artery

3-62

Removal of Fragments in Circumferential Fashion—Right Carotid Exposure

Before beginning the repair of the arteriotomy, it is necessary to inspect the bed of the carotid plaque for any loose fragments that might need to be removed. Failure to attend to this detail may result in free fragments of material in the arterial lumen, which can create the nidus for thrombus formation and subsequent embolization. I prefer to gently stroke the denuded area with a small peanut sponge, which brings up any loose edges, particularly if the stroking is done in a caudad to cephalad direction. Fragments should be grasped with the vascular forceps and peeled off in circumferential fashion. If the removal process is begun either in the center of the vessel or on one edge, the fragment will peel off in a circular fashion until it reaches the other edge of the arteriotomy. It is important to avoid further traumatizing of the denuded area.

Areas of retained intima that are solidly attached to the vessel wall need not be dissected free. Only areas with a loose edge and which readily submit to circumferential removal need be scrupulously eliminated from the arterial bed.

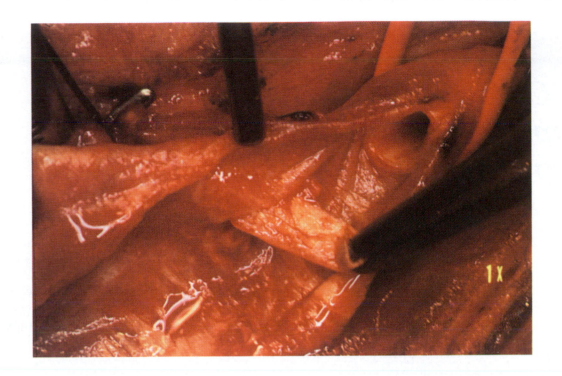

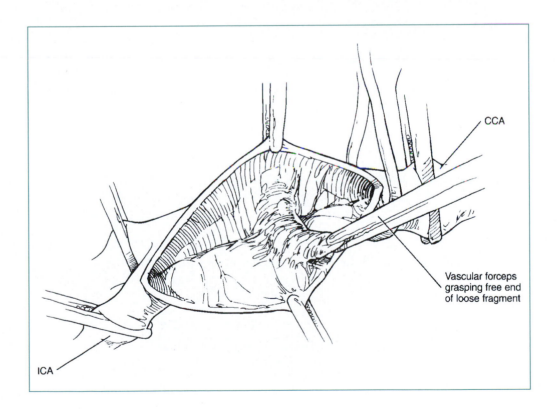

CCA

Vascular forceps
grasping free end
of loose fragment

ICA

3-63

Left Carotid Endarterectomy— Completed Removal, Sharp Margins

After completed removal of the plaque from the internal, common, and external carotid arteries, a denuded area of vessel wall is seen and the arteriotomy is ready for arterial repair to begin. In this figure, note the sharp margin where the normal shelf of intima begins in the ICA. Whether this particular example would require a tacking stitch would depend on how it responded to palpation and whether the surgeon believed it represented a loose edge. The yellow area of the sharp removal of plaque can be seen peeking out from the arteriotomy edge at the CCA as well. Once the fragments have been removed in circumferential fashion, the vessel is ready for arterial repair, which begins distally in the ICA.

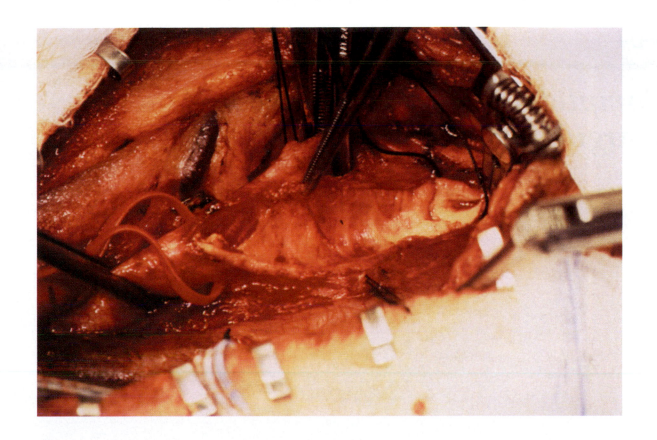

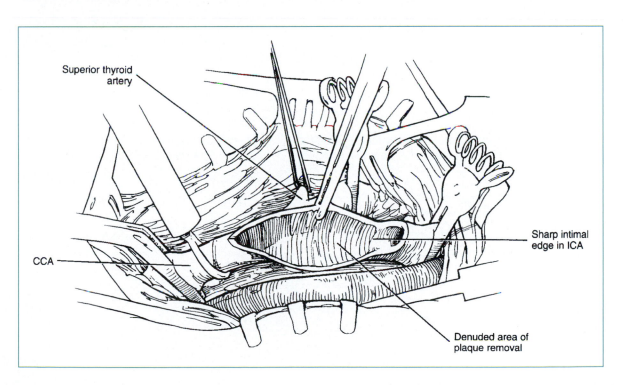

Superior thyroid artery

CCA

Sharp intimal edge in ICA

Denuded area of plaque removal

3-64

Completed Removal, Sharp Margins—Left Carotid Exposure

A second example shows a somewhat closer view of a sharp margin after removal of the plaque in its entirety from the common, internal, and external carotid arteries. In this particular case, the plaque is feathered nicely from the ICA and there is no visible need to place tacking sutures. All fragments appear to have been removed, and the vessel is ready for surgical repair of the arteriotomy.

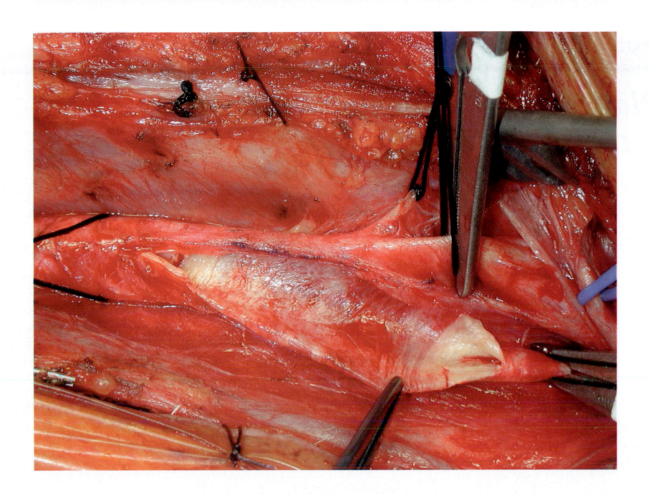

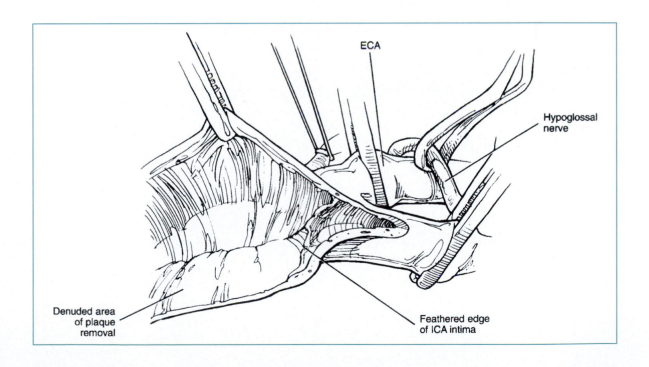

ECA

Hypoglossal
nerve

Denuded area
of plaque
removal

Feathered edge
of ICA intima

3-65

Placement of Tacking Sutures in Internal Carotid Artery

As mentioned, I do my best to follow the atheroma up high enough in the ICA, so that it feathers completely, leaving a smooth transition zone without the need for tacking sutures. However, there is no question in my mind that in perhaps 10% to 20% of cases I am dissatisfied with the transition zone and I believe that tacking sutures should be placed.

When this is necessary, I try to place tacking sutures in three positions in the circumference of the arterial wall. They are placed posteriorly at the four and eight o'clock positions, and the third is a de facto tacking suture placed by picking up all levels of the vessel wall in the repaired arterial suture line at essentially 12 o'clock position. The sutures are double-armed 6-0 Prolene that are passed from the inside out to cross the shelf of the intimal edge. The knot can then be tied outside the vessel wall so that no thrombogenic knot or loose end is left within the vessel lumen. It is important to place these sutures accurately because once they are tied, it is essentially impossible to remove them. Gently stroking with a peanut sponge will then indicate whether the loose flap has been adequately secured.

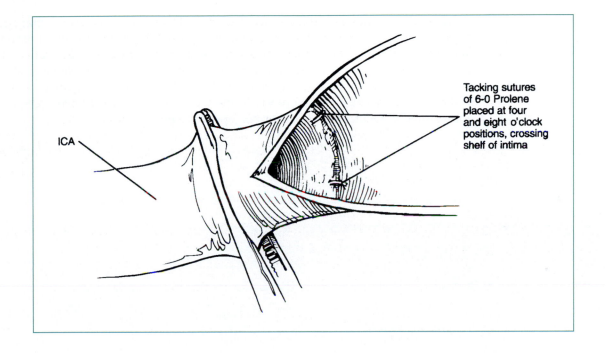

ICA

Tacking sutures
of 6-0 Prolene
placed at four
and eight o'clock
positions, crossing
shelf of intima

3-66

Anatomic Variant—Atherosclerotic Web on Posterior Wall of Vessel

On several occasions I have identified regions of thrombus and stenosis that appear to originate from a posterior atherosclerotic shelf protruding into the lumen of the vessel from the back wall. These have sometimes been persistent even after removal of the atheroma. In cases such as this my strategy has been to place a single vertical stitch in the same fashion as a tacking suture to hold this shelf down flat against the back wall of the vessel. This has worked nicely in the few cases in which I have used it and has not resulted in recurrent stenosis or postoperative thrombosis.

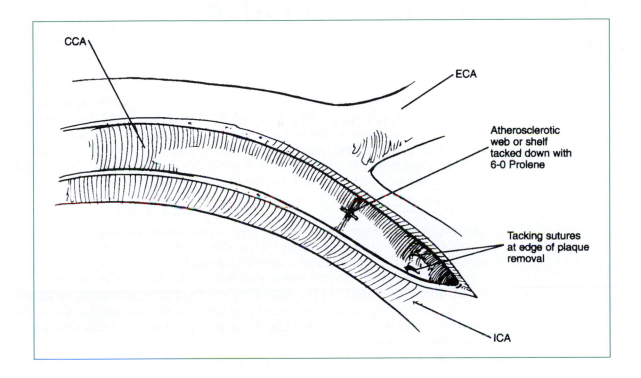

3-67

Repair Beginning in Internal Carotid Artery—Left Carotid Exposure—No Patch Graft

When all fragments have been removed from the arterial bed, the repair begins in the distal ICA. A single anchor bite is placed distal to the apex of the arteriotomy and secured with a surgeon's knot followed by nine more throws. Tiny bites are then taken in continuous, nonlocking fashion approximately 1 mm back from the arteriotomy edge and approximately 1 to 2 mm apart. It is extremely important that the ICA portion of the repair be done with fine bites, and some authors advocate the use of the microscope for this purpose. I believe the repair can be satisfactorily performed under magnified (×3.5) loupe vision, and the experienced surgeon is not likely to encounter inadvertent stenosis. Deep or large bites in the ICA repair may create an area of focal stenosis that would be thrombogenic. As can be seen in this figure, the suture line is brought down to the region of the carotid bulb where the lumen becomes much wider. At this point, somewhat larger bites may be taken. A second suture line is begun in the CCA where a broad, deep bite is taken just proximal to the crotch of the arteriotomy and likewise continuous, nonlocking sutures are brought up until the first suture line is met. When the two sutures meet and can be tied together at the center of the incision, the artery is prepared for final closure.

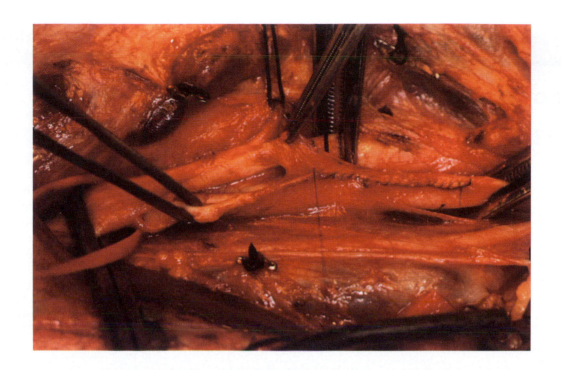

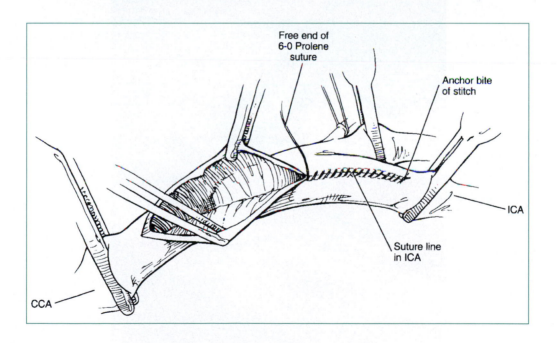

3-68

Microscopic Internal Carotid Artery Repair

As mentioned previously in the text, I stopped using the operating microscope for carotid repair when I adopted a strategy of universal roof patch grafting. This photograph shows an older case of mine and the extremely fine ICA repair that is possible under the microscope, and many of my colleagues continue to value this surgical approach. In this case the 6-0 Prolene repair on the ICA is almost invisible to the unaided eye when the microscope has been removed. The bulldog clamp is on the ECA.

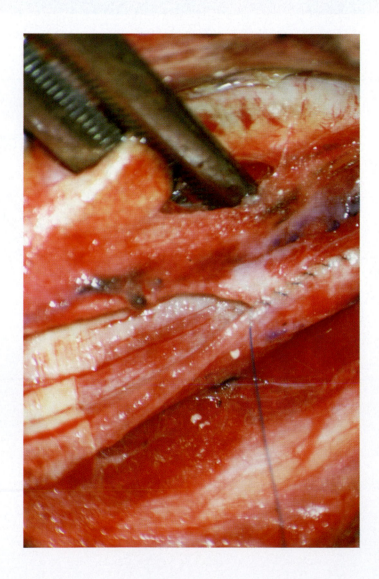

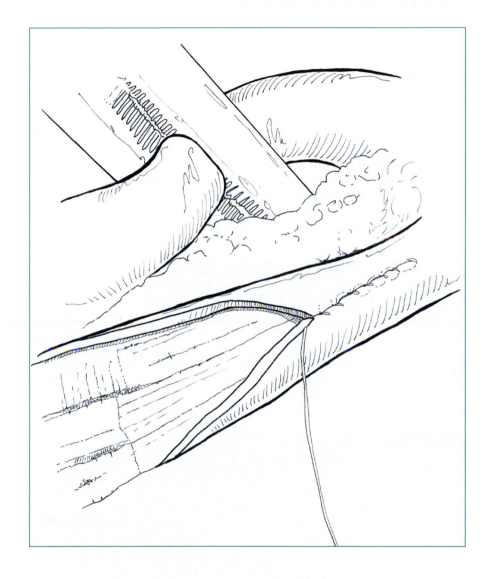

3-69

Repair Beginning in External Carotid Artery—Right Carotid Exposure—No Patch Graft

When it is necessary to open the ECA endarterectomy as a separate Y-shaped incision as previously mentioned, I prefer to begin by repairing the ECA arteriotomy first. An anchor stitch is placed distal to the apex of the ECA arteriotomy, and working distally to proximally, a continuous interrupted nonlocking suture is placed. At the carotid bulb, a separate single stitch is thrown and tied, and the free end of the continuous ECA stitch is tied to this. The other free end of the single stitch can then be incorporated into the main arteriotomy suture line. This figure demonstrates a complete ECA repair.

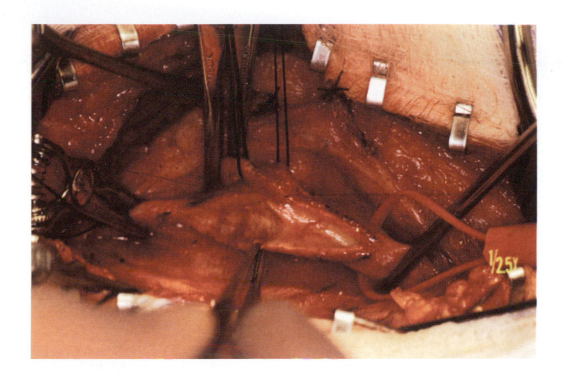

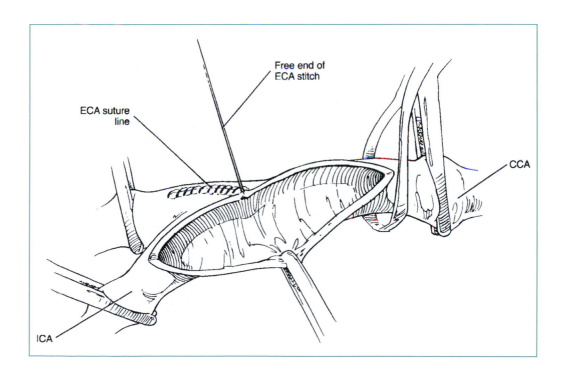

Free end of
ECA stitch

ECA suture
line

CCA

ICA

3-70

Repair of External Carotid Artery—Left Carotid Exposure—No Patch Graft

A somewhat closer view of a completed ECA repair in a left CEA is shown. The open lumen of the common and internal carotid arteries following endarterectomy is readily seen. The anchor stitch was placed in the distal ECA; a continuous suture was brought down to the region of the carotid bulb over the free end, and the ECA stitch is visible. The tie securing the ECA stitch is also evident at the region of the carotid bulb. The repair of the ICA now begins and later will be brought together with the repair in the CCA.

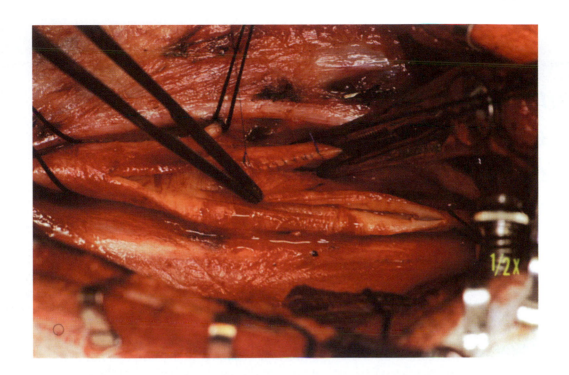

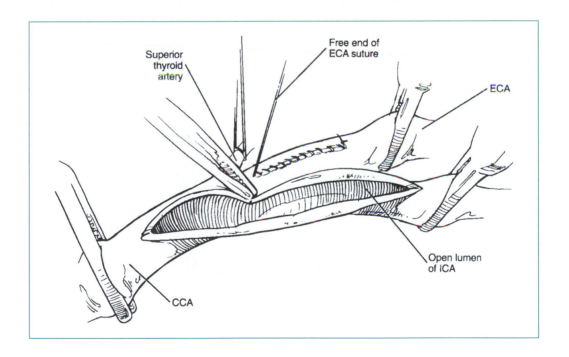

Superior thyroid artery

Free end of ECA suture

ECA

CCA

Open lumen of ICA

3-71

Second Limb of Repair Coming Up Common Carotid Artery— No Patch Graft

When the ICA suture line has been brought down to the region of the carotid bulb, the 6-0 Prolene is secured with a rubber-shod mosquito clamp and draped away from the field. A second arm of the suture line is brought up from the CCA. This begins by taking a large full-thickness bite proximal to the apex of the arteriotomy in the CCA. The same type of equal bites are then taken to create a suture line that comes up until it meets the ICA suture line in the region of the carotid bulb. The bites in the CCA need not be as fine because the potential for creating a stenosis is much less. I customarily have the CCA suture line performed by the assistant since a right-handed assistant will place the bites from right to left just as the primary surgeon did in the ICA. In this way, the needles will come out on opposite sides of the vessel at the carotid bulb and the knot will lie across the arteriotomy wall rather than having both stitches on the same side. I think this is important to secure adequate hemostasis at the point where the two suture lines are brought together.

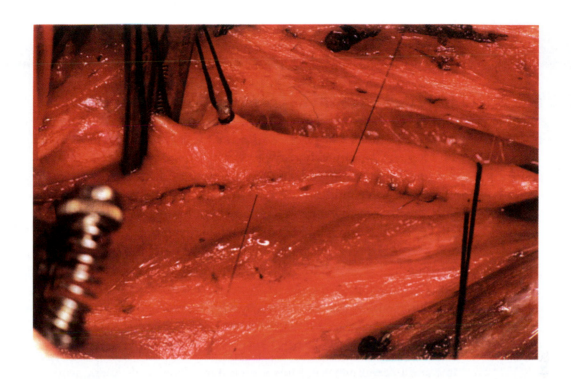

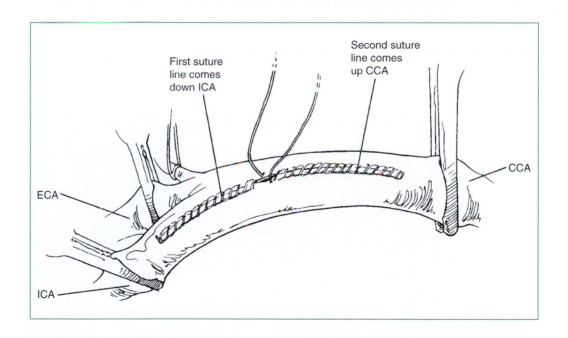

First suture
line comes
down ICA

Second suture
line comes
up CCA

CCA

ECA

ICA

3-72

Suture Sequence and Placement of the Hemashield Roof Patch Graft on the Internal Carotid Artery

This series of photographs shows my design for a hemostatic and patent placement of the roof patch graft. The graft is first tapered at both ends with scissors, then anchored at both ends, as shown in (A) with inside-out sutures of double-armed 6-0 Prolene, taking special care to be certain that the bites on the CCA and ICA are deep, firm, and solid. I then proceed to suture the medial wall from ICA to ECA, taking bites with loupe-magnified vision that are approximately 1 mm deep on both sides and 1mm apart, using a running, non-locking stitch, as show in (B). The loose end of this medial wall stitch is tied to one of the ends of the CCA anchor stitch with 10 knots. One is then able to peek at the inside of the vessel, shown in (C), to confirm the integrity of the suture line and to ensure that no clots have formed. Finally the lateral wall is closed by using the second arm of the ICA anchor stitch to come halfway down the lateral wall (D), where the stitch will ultimately be tied to a second arm which comes halfway up from the ICA (not illustrated).

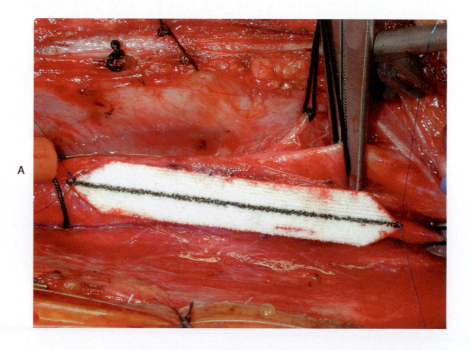

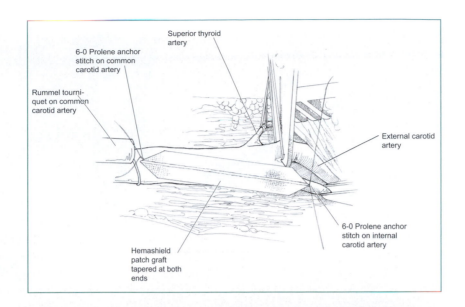

Superior thyroid artery

6-0 Prolene anchor stitch on common carotid artery

Rummel tourniquet on common carotid artery

External carotid artery

6-0 Prolene anchor stitch on internal carotid artery

Hemashield patch graft tapered at both ends

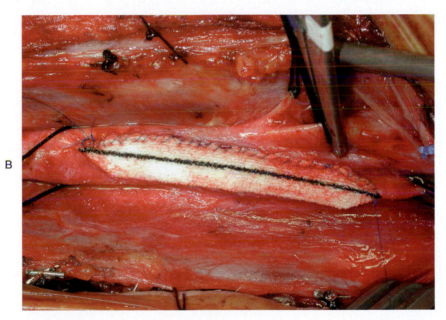

B

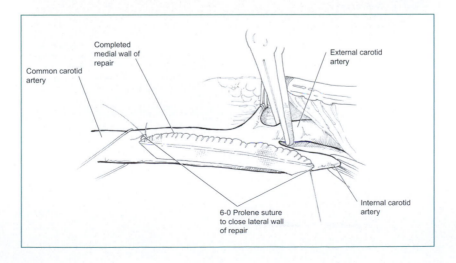

Completed medial wall of repair

Common carotid artery

External carotid artery

6-0 Prolene suture to close lateral wall of repair

Internal carotid artery

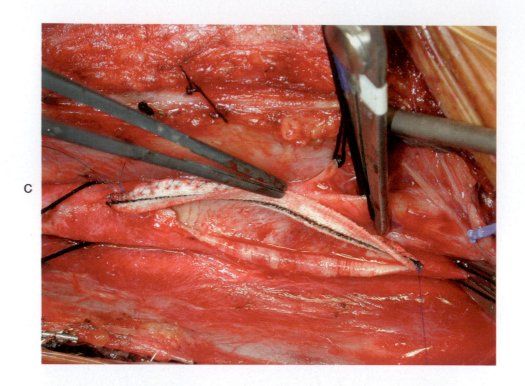

C

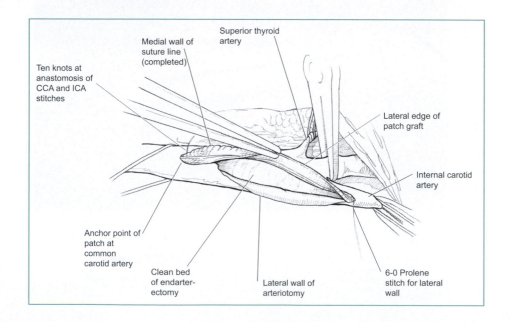

Ten knots at
anastomosis of
CCA and ICA
stitches

Medial wall of
suture line
(completed)

Superior thyroid
artery

Lateral edge of
patch graft

Internal carotid
artery

Anchor point of
patch at
common
carotid artery

Clean bed
of endarter-
ectomy

Lateral wall of
arteriotomy

6-0 Prolene
stitch for lateral
wall

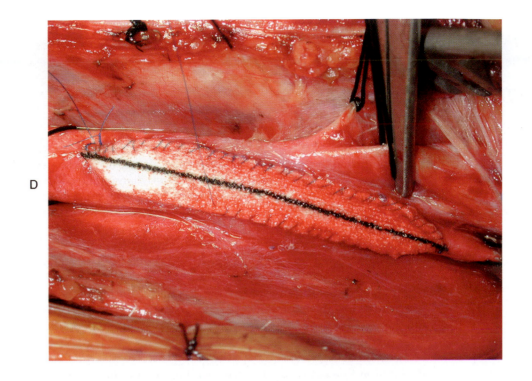

D

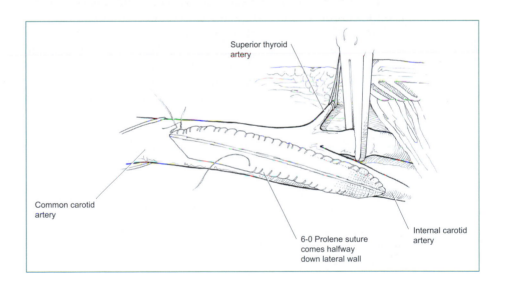

Superior thyroid
artery

Common carotid
artery

6-0 Prolene suture
comes halfway
down lateral wall

Internal carotid
artery

3-73

Removal of Shunt

When a shunt has been used, it will be necessary to remove it before final closure of the vessel. I do this in the following fashion. When there is approximately 1 cm of open vessel remaining, I use two small straight mosquito clamps introduced within the lumen to clamp the shunt closed with approximately 5 mm of open shunt between them. I then use straight scissors to cut the shunt in half, being certain to ensure that I do not cut the back wall in the process. The Javid or Loftus clamp is then removed from the ICA, and the distal end of the shunt is slid back and removed from the wound. A bulldog clamp is quickly reapplied to minimize backbleeding. The CCA end of the shunt is then removed by pulling it up out of the lumen at the carotid bulb. It is not necessary to significantly loosen the Rummel tourniquet to remove the shunt; doing so promotes bleeding. Once the shunt has been removed from the CCA, the DeBakey cross-clamp is immediately applied to minimize antegrade bleeding and the Rummel tourniquet is released completely. The most common error in shunt removal is to entangle the Prolene in the straight mosquito clamps used to double clamp the shunt. One must take great caution to ensure that this does not happen because Prolene tangled in the mosquito clamp will hamper removal of the cut shunt at exactly the worst possible time.

This process must proceed quickly. The patient is ischemic during shunt removal since the carotid tree is completely closed and the monitoring system—whether EEG, TCD, or SSEP—-will most likely demonstrate ischemia once again. The standard measurement for ischemic time during shunt removal and completion of repair is five minutes, but in my experience it customarily takes a minute or two less.

Once the shunt has been removed, the needle is picked up from one end of the suture line (usually the internal since the primary surgeon will most likely be performing this step) and I proceed to finish with the closure of the vessel. The final evacuation of air, backbleeding, and filling of the vessel with heparin saline are performed in the same fashion as will be described for cases in which a shunt has not been used.

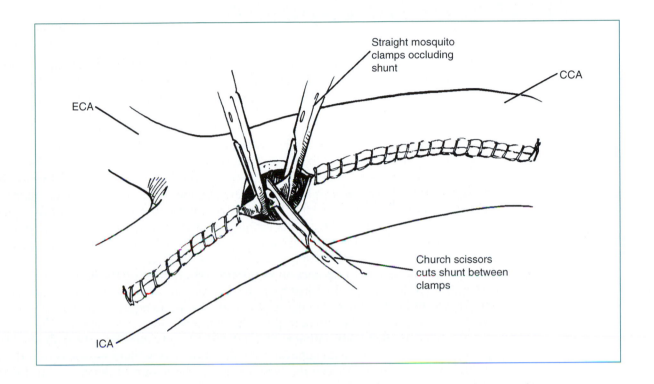

Straight mosquito
clamps occluding
shunt

CCA

ECA

Church scissors
cuts shunt between
clamps

ICA

3-74

Tying Together—Evacuation of Air—Right Carotid Exposure

A rigid protocol must be followed for the reconstitution of flow in the clamped carotid tree. When the suture line is completed in the ICA, a second suture line comes up the CCA. These suture lines meet in the region of the carotid bulb and are eventually tied together. First, however, all three vessels are backbled, usually in the sequence of internal, external, and common carotid arteries. I hold a finger over the suture line to prevent blood from spraying the surgeon's or assistant's face when the CCA is briefly opened. With a little practice, no more than 1 or 2 mL should escape during this process. When the vessels have been backbled and it is clear that no thrombosis of a distal vessel has occurred or inadvertent stenosis has been created by the suture line, the vessels are ready for final closure. On rare occasions, ICA backbleeding will be inadequate; this is most often a consequence of having a 0 silk string pulled taut by a mosquito clamp, holding the vessel closed even when the bulldog clamp has been released. With gentle relaxation of this occluding silk, backbleeding usually ensues. In a case of true backbleeding failure, it may be necessary to advance an exploratory shunt tube up the ICA, drawing back with suction to reestablish flow, just as in the case of complete thrombosis of the carotid tree. This technique is illustrated in Fig. 4-2. Failing this, a Fogarty catheter also may be used to reestablish flow. Fortunately, this is an extremely rare occurrence.

When adequate backbleeding is ensured and air and debris have been flushed free by this process, a syringe with heparinized saline and a long blunt needle is introduced into the arterial lumen between the two stitches in the region of the carotid bulb. The stitches are held taut by the primary surgeon, and a surgeon's knot is thrown but not drawn tight. The lumen is then filled with heparinized saline until the carotid tree bulges. As this filling process is taking place, all final air and debris are expelled and the surgeon's knot is taken down to secure the two stitches. I then use nine more single throws to ensure an adequate closure.

Occasionally, a large leak develops from the pressure of the heparin saline infusion. At this point I stop, throw a single stitch across the point of leakage, and continue to close the vessel in the same fashion, repeating the heparinized saline flushing step.

When all the knots are thrown, the ends of the stitches are left long; if a leak occurs in the region of the carotid bulb, it can then be controlled by taking another bite with the attached needle and retying.

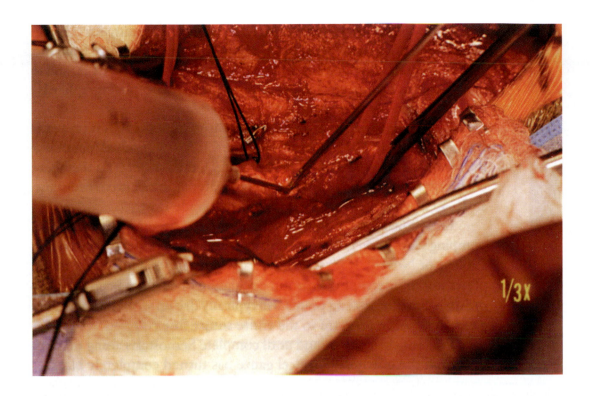

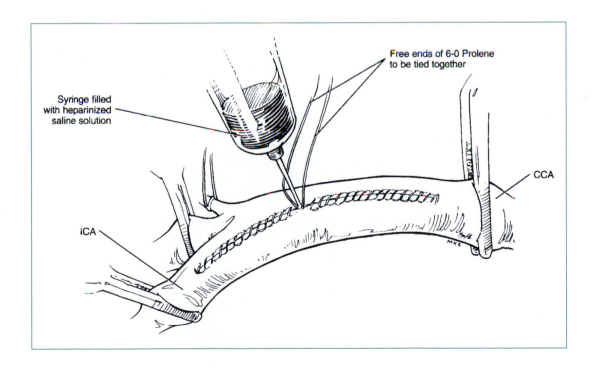

Syringe filled with heparinized saline solution

Free ends of 6-0 Prolene to be tied together

CCA

ICA

3-75

Blunt Needle to Evacuate Air and Debris as Final Step— Patch Graft

Here is an even better illustration of the blunt needle evacuation technique in a case with a Hemashield roof patch. One can appreciate that a small opening is left at the midpoint of the lateral wall. After back-bleeding all three vessels, the heparinized saline in the syringe is slowly infused by the assistant, filling the vessel while the primary surgeon ties both sutures together, after which the needle is withdrawn. Needless to say, we do not tie the sutures until the runback is pure saline, without air bubbles or debris.

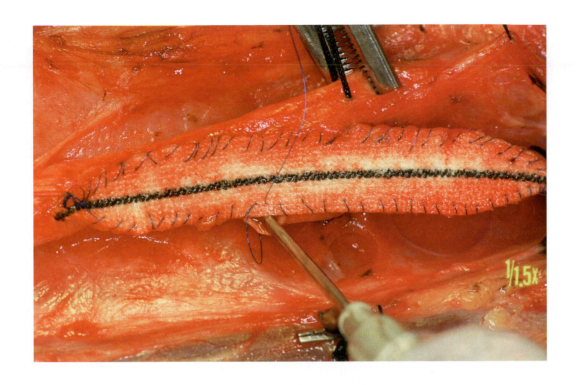

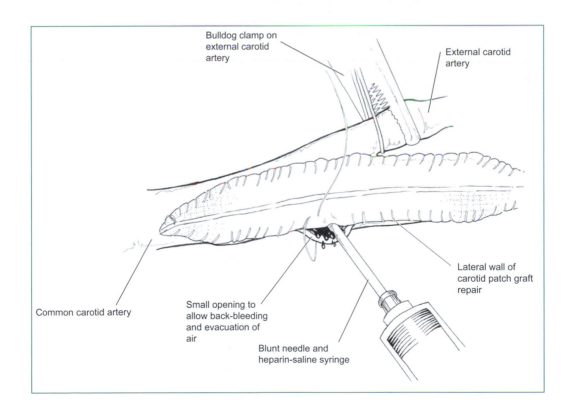

Bulldog clamp on
external carotid
artery

External carotid
artery

Lateral wall of
carotid patch graft
repair

Common carotid artery

Small opening to
allow back-bleeding
and evacuation of
air

Blunt needle and
heparin-saline syringe

3-76

Sequence of Clamp Removal at Completion of Arteriotomy

Once the vessel has been completely closed, it is ready for clamp removal. I remove the clamp first from the ECA, and immediately afterward from the CCA. I then wait 10 seconds, allowing any air and debris to flush up the ECA, and then I remove the ICA cross clamp, after which time the electroencephalographer is notified that the circulation has been restored.

The purpose of this procedure is to ensure that the ICA is protected at all times. By opening the ECA followed first by the CCA, any residual material will flush into the face, where it will be of no consequence. Until I am certain that there is no potential for untoward embolization of foreign material, under no circumstances will I open an ICA clamp and expose the brain to antegrade flow.

Occasional leaks along the suture line may become evident at this point. *Frank* pumping leaks often need to be repaired with an accurately placed single stitch of 6-0 Prolene. It is rarely necessary to reapply clamps to accomplish this, and I prefer not to interrupt the carotid circulation once it has been reestablished, if at all possible. Smaller, oozing points will typically dry up with the application of Surgicel gauze and gentle pressure to the entire suture line.

I do not close the wound until complete hemostasis along the suture line is ensured and the overlying Surgicel gauze has turned completely black.

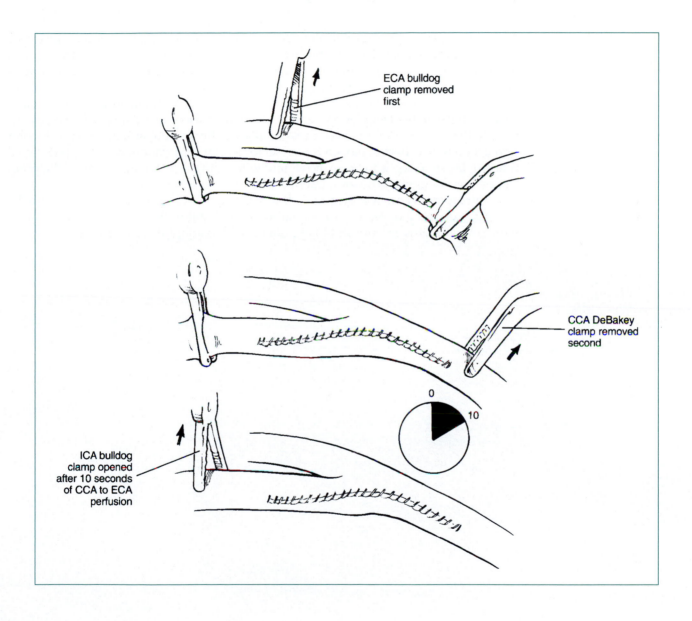

ECA bulldog
clamp removed
first

CCA DeBakey
clamp removed
second

ICA bulldog
clamp opened
after 10 seconds
of CCA to ECA
perfusion

3-77

Doppler Examination of Repair—Left Carotid Exposure

A Doppler probe examination of all three branches of the carotid tree verifies adequacy of the surgical repair. The carotid artery has been completely closed, the clamps removed, and hemostasis achieved. Audible patency provides early reassurance until a neurologic examination is possible.

Common causes of failure to auscultate the Doppler signal include broken probes, weak batteries in the Doppler box, and inadequate moistness of the vessel being examined. In the rare instance in which these details are checked but still there is no Doppler signal, I do not hesitate to reopen the vessel for a brief exploration. If no Doppler signal is heard, the first step is to flood the wound with saline, which usually solves the problem by improving the acoustical interface between vessel and probe.

Intraoperative angiography and ultrasound have been described for evaluating the technical adequacy of repair or eliminating the possibility of thrombosis. Fortunately, these complications are rare and I have not needed to adopt these techniques.

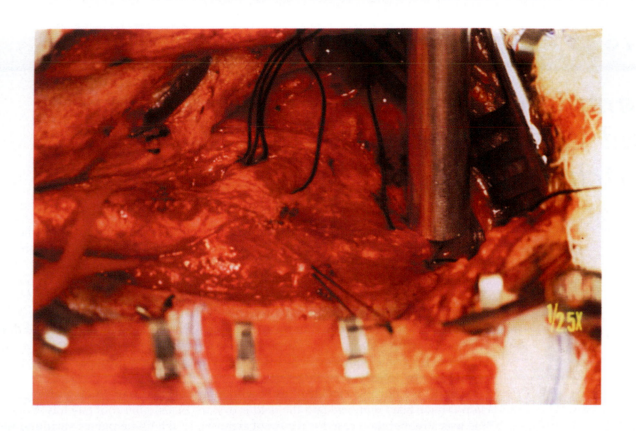

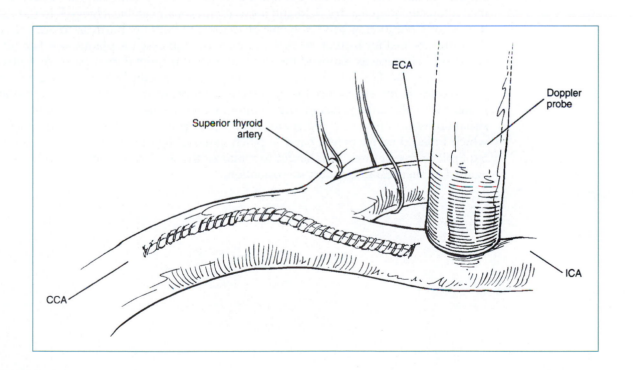

3-78

Completed Dry Repair Without and With Hemashield Patch Graft

Four examples of the completed dry suture line prior to closure of the carotid sheath are shown. As previously mentioned, I do not close the carotid sheath when there is any evidence whatsoever of bleeding from the arteriotomy site. Keep in mind that the arterial repair is typically evaluated in light of either normal or hypertensive blood pressure. If the patient is hypotensive, I ask the anesthesiologist to elevate blood pressure at least to baseline levels in order to thoroughly evaluate the repair.

Surgicel was not applied to the suture line in these cases, but I do like to line the arteriotomy with a long strip of Surgicel gauze in every case prior to closing the sheath. Likewise, I place a Hemovac, which is removed on the first postoperative day, in the carotid sheath directly over the artery.

In (E) we illustrate an ideal result with a Hemashield roof patch graft repair. The clamps have been removed and the field is dry. In (F) a similar roof patch is shown, but this was a reoperation case for recurrent stenosis, so the tissue planes surrounding the carotid sheath vessels are blurred and indistinct. Clearly with careful dissection and meticulous technique a dry field and a successful repair can be achieved. In (G) I show the use of a reinforcing band of hemashield graft material to buttress an area of vessel thinning (see text for further details). In this particular case the plaque was heavily calcified, and after it was removed the residual wall was quite thin in parts. As I placed a single stitch to stop a small leak after declamping, the needle hole enlarged and continued to ooze. In my experience the placement of more sutures would have compounded rather than solved the problem. My solution, which we use occasionally in this type of situation, was to first stop the oozing with direct pressure, which was effective, after which I placed an encircling band of patch material tied together at the top with two 6-0 Prolene-free sutures. This serves to reinforce the weak area and hopefully to guard against further leaks or aneurysm formation.

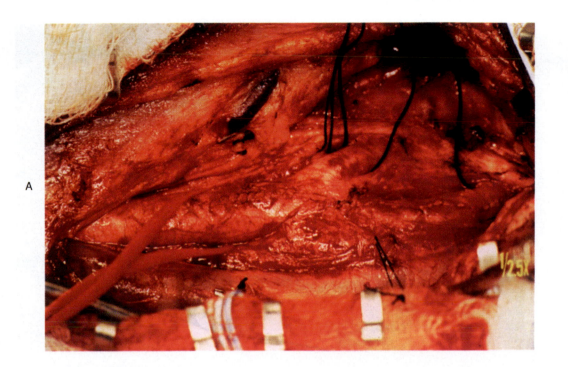

A

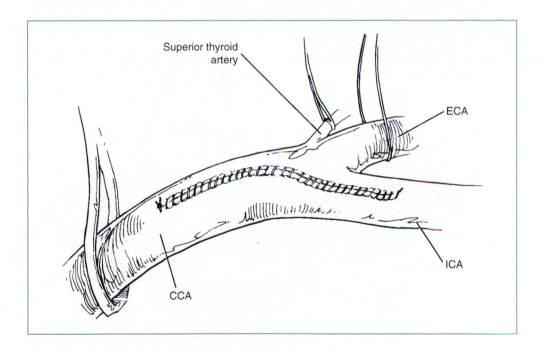

Superior thyroid artery

ECA

ICA

CCA

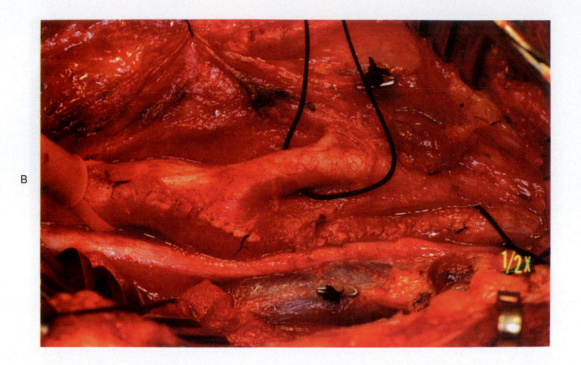

B

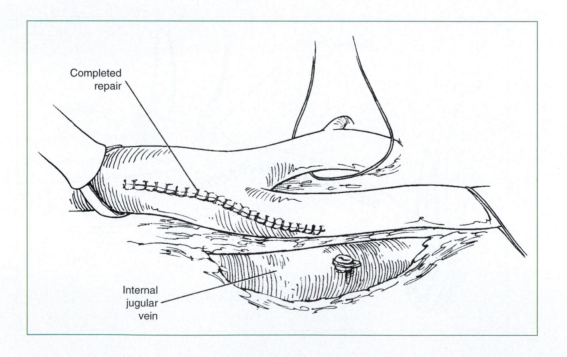

Completed repair

Internal jugular vein

C

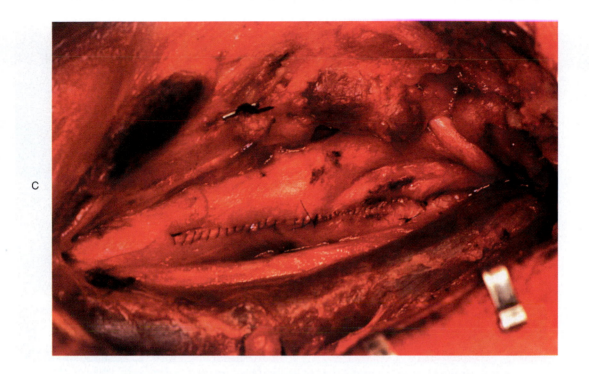

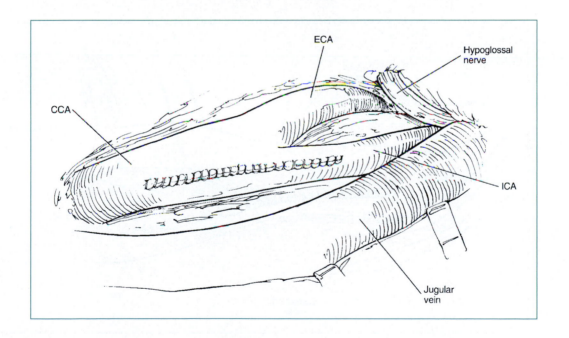

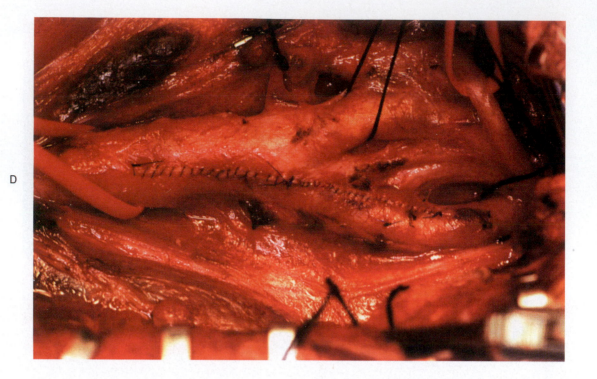

D

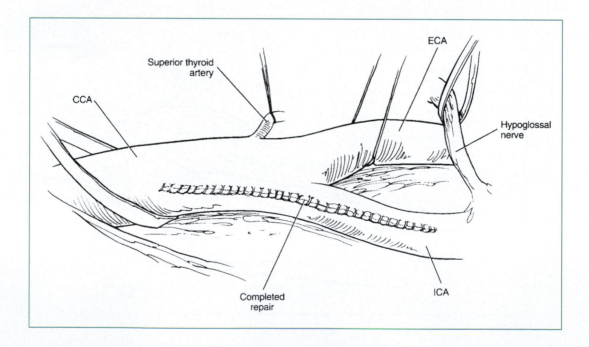

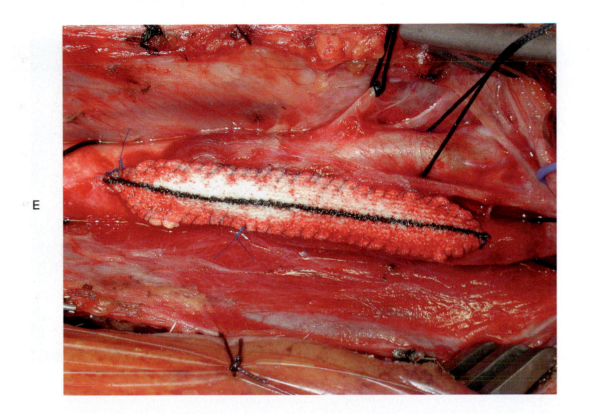

E

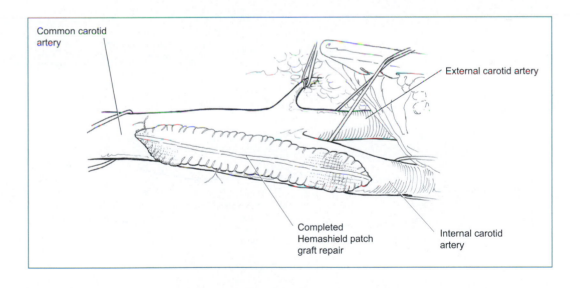

Common carotid
artery

External carotid artery

Completed
Hemashield patch
graft repair

Internal carotid
artery

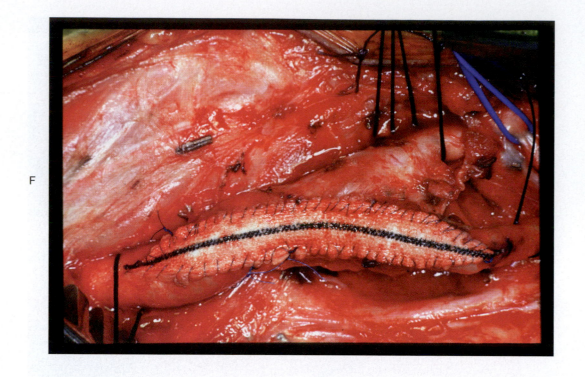

F

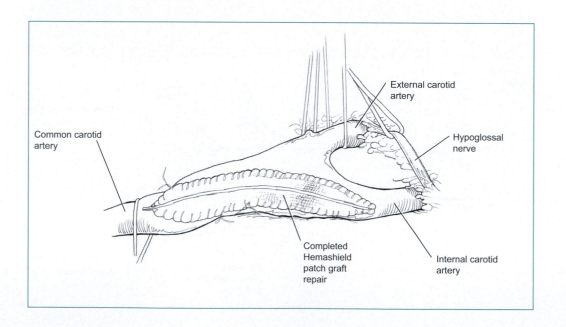

Common carotid
artery

External carotid
artery

Hypoglossal
nerve

Completed
Hemashield
patch graft
repair

Internal carotid
artery

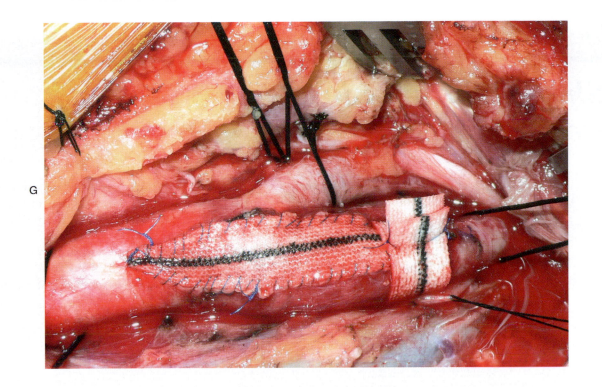

G

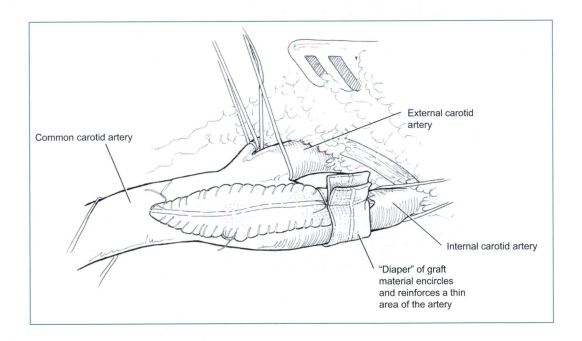

Common carotid artery

External carotid artery

Internal carotid artery

"Diaper" of graft material encircles and reinforces a thin area of the artery

3-79

Y-Shaped Suture Line—No Patch Graft

This is a right CEA in which a separate ECA endarterectomy and repair were performed. The Y-shaped suture line of 6-0 Prolene can be seen; note the convergence of the external and internal carotid repairs at the region of the carotid bulb. When blood flow is reestablished, it is common for the ICA repair to rotate with the reopening of the vessel. In this case, the ICA suture line was straight up the midportion of the vessel when the arteriotomy was performed. Later, the repair rotated because dissection of the lateral attachments of the carotid bed is always more extensive than that medial to the carotid bifurcation.

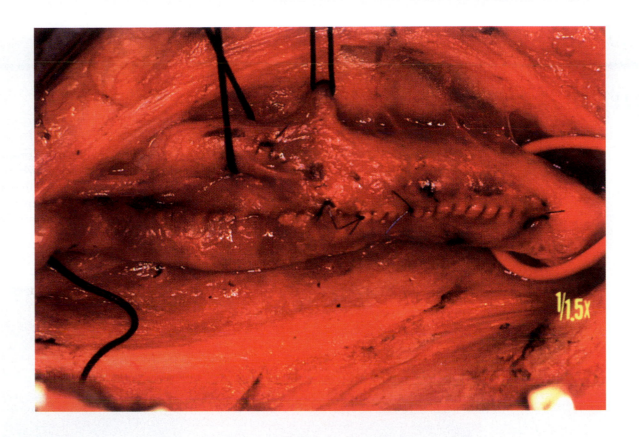

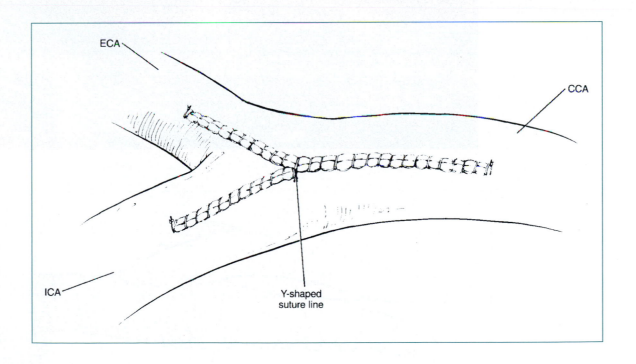

3-80

Surgicel on Dry Repair

This figure demonstrates the placement of Surgicel along the suture line of a non-patch case (A), which I customarily do when the repair is assessed to be dry. When the Surgicel turns black, as seen in this figure, there is certain to be no further active arterial bleeding and closure of the wound can begin after placement of the Hemovac.

In (B), we have applied Surgicel gauze over a Hemashield patch graft repair. There is essentially no bleeding here, so the gauze remains white in this illustration.

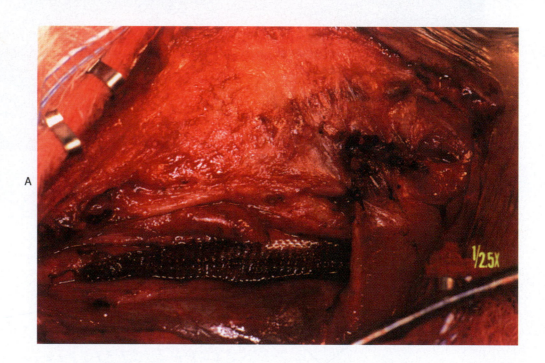

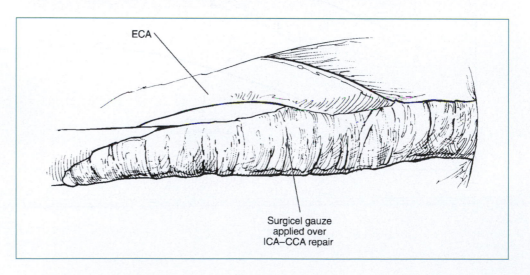

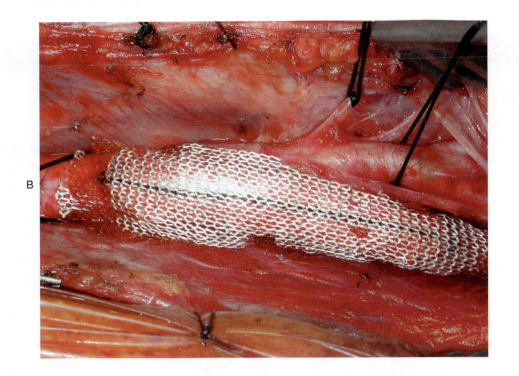

B

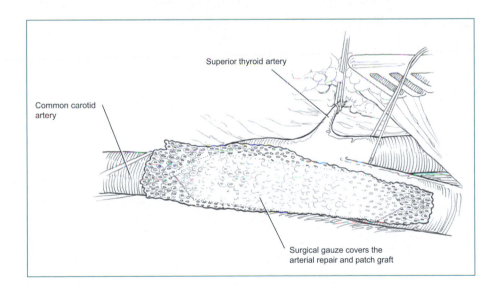

Superior thyroid artery

Common carotid
artery

Surgical gauze covers the
arterial repair and patch graft

3-81

Closure of Sheath

The carotid sheath is reopposed by pulling up the sternocleidomastoid muscle to some medial fascia and closing this layer with interrupted sutures of 3-0 Vicryl placed approximately 1 cm apart. This closure of the shealth is an important layer, both to secure the Hemovac and to prevent infection. In one case I encountered a superficial wound infection that fortunately respected this layer of the closed carotid sheath and did not penetrate to deeper structures.

It is important to remember that nerves can be damaged by deep bites on the medial side; deep bites on the lateral side under the sternocleidomastoid muscle also could injure the jugular vein. The rule is to place superficial bites on both the sternocleidomastoid edge and along the medial fascia. Likewise, it is important to remember the area where the common facial vein was ligated so that a needle is not inadvertently placed through the distal stump.

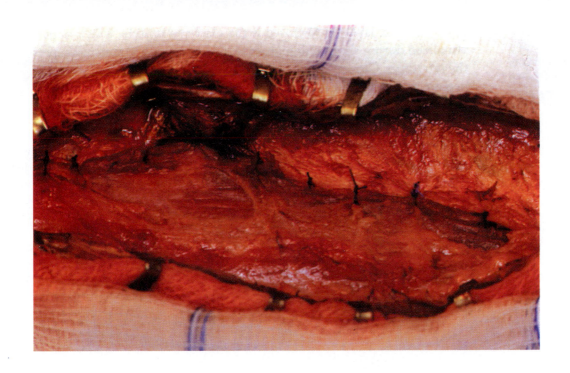

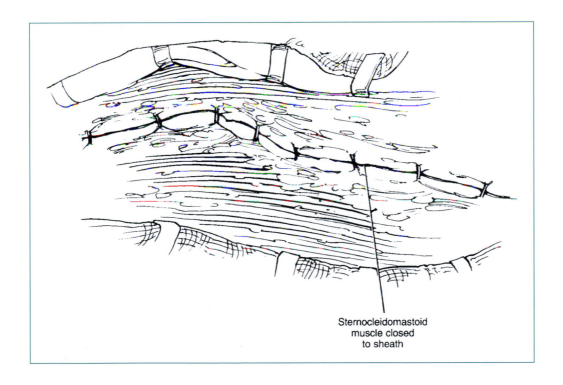

Sternocleidomastoid
muscle closed
to sheath

3-82

Closure of Platysma

The next layer to be closed is the platysma muscle, which hopefully was well visualized during the opening process and has remained somewhat preserved under the retractors. Closure of the platysma yields a nice cosmetic result on the neck; even in patients with a vertical incision, the surgical wound is nearly invisible after six months. I attribute the improved cosmetic result to scrupulous repair of the platysma muscle, preventing tension along skin lines.

Note that the Michel clips are left on the wound until after the platysma is closed. I find that Michel clips and wound edge sponges help prevent the troublesome wound edge bleeding that often occurs while the platysma is being closed. For this reason, care is taken at the beginning of the procedure to ensure that the platysma is not included in the Michel clips.

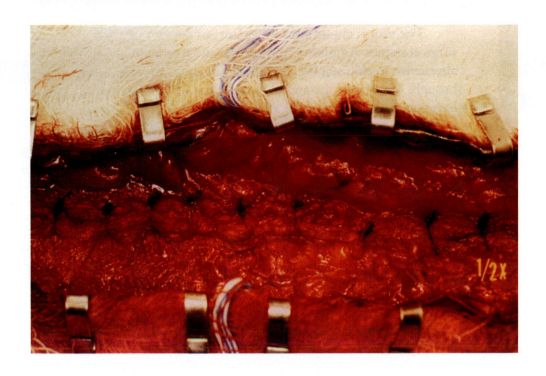

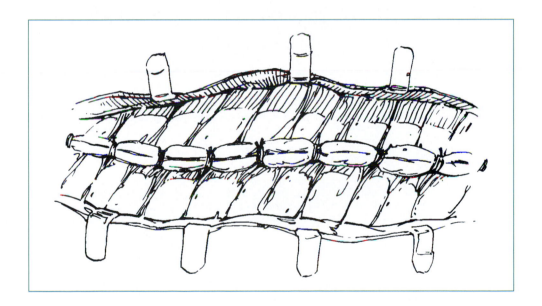

3-83

Skin and Hemovac

The skin is closed with subcutaneous stitches of 3-0 or 4-0 Vicryl followed by a running subcuticular stitch of undyed 4-0 Vicryl. The Hemovac drain that lies inside the carotid sheath is brought out, always through the caudal end of the wound and with care taken not to harpoon the external jugular vein in the process. As mentioned, the Hemovac drain is placed to canister suction only and is removed on the first postoperative day. I have found that the use of the Hemovac drain prevents the large ecchymotic neck frequently associated with subcutaneous dissection of minor wound bleeding. In my patients, the heparin is not reversed intraoperatively and they are placed back on their aspirin regimens immediately after surgery.

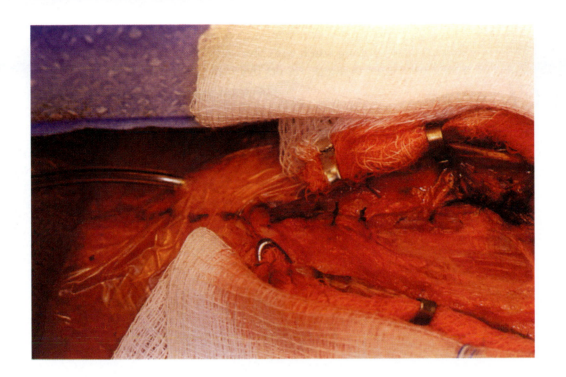

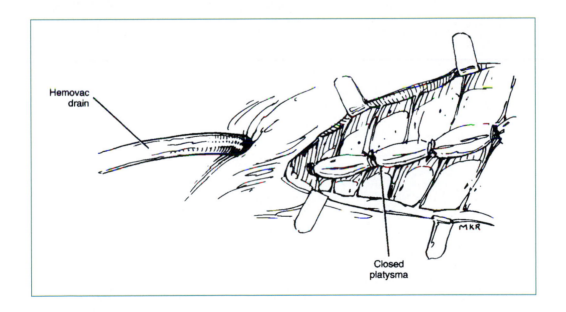

Hemovac
drain

Closed
platysma

3-84

Skin Closure

We now close carotid incisions with a running subcuticular stitch and dermabond adhesive to anneal the skin edges, which allows the patient to cleanse the wound and provides an excellent cosmetic result as the sutures dissolve and the skin flattens out. The incision is barely visible after 6 months, despite my preference for a vertical sternomastoid based incision rather than a horizontal skin crease type opening.

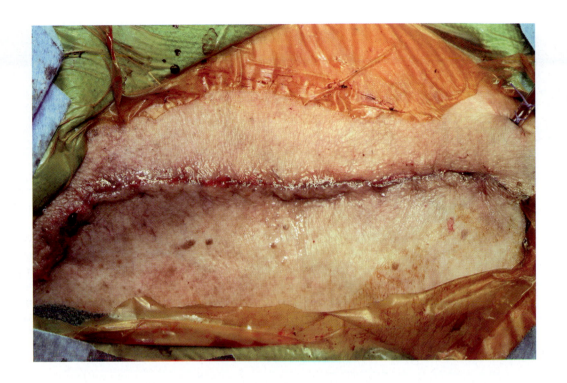

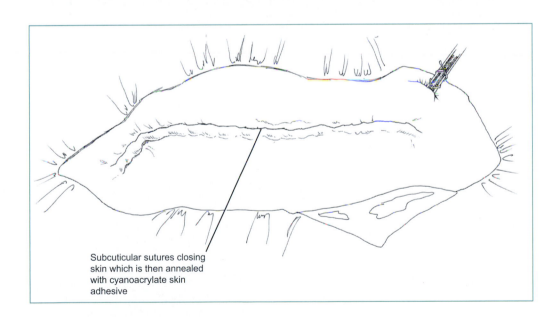

Subcuticular sutures closing skin which is then annealed with cyanoacrylate skin adhesive

3-85

Placement of Saphenous Vein Patch Graft

For the sake of completeness, I included this illustration of a saphenous vein patch graft. I no longer use this technique, and have converted entirely to the Hemashield graft material.

The technique is simple whether the case is shunted or unshunted. An elliptic-shaped patch graft is fashioned from high saphenous vein and oriented so that there will be no valves to impede the column of flow. An anchor bite is then placed in the ICA, and a long suture line is run along the medial aspect of the repair. The lateral aspect of the repair is closed with a two-armed suture line, just as in a primary carotid repair, facilitating evacuation of the intraluminal contents prior to final closure and likewise facilitating removal of the shunt if a shunt has been called for by monitoring parameters.

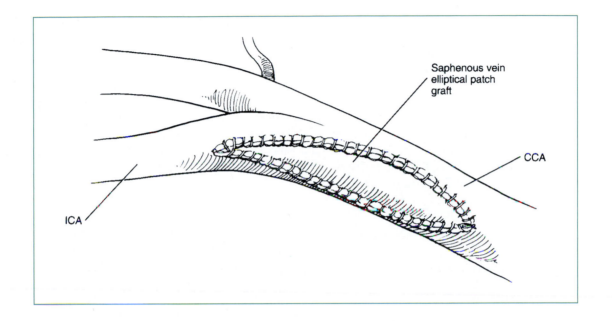

Saphenous vein
elliptical patch
graft

CCA

ICA

CHAPTER 4

Complications

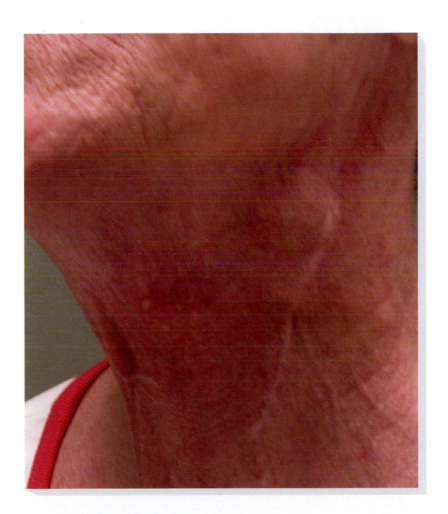

4-1

Acute Postoperative Internal Carotid Artery Thrombosis

This is a major complication of carotid endarterectomy. It is also an old case, which predates my adoption of the universal patch graft strategy. This patient had a primary (not patched) right sided CCA to ICA repair without problems. She became marginally hypotensive in the post-anesthesia recovery area and developed a mild to moderate left-sided hemiparesis. We took her quickly to angiography where an acute occlusion was documented. I returned her immediately to surgery for re-exploration and revision with roof patch graft. I could not identify a technical error that accounted for the thrombosis, and in my mind it was explained by the combination of hypotension, a diabetic patient, and a female with a small internal carotid artery. Fortunately she made a complete recovery following her second operation.

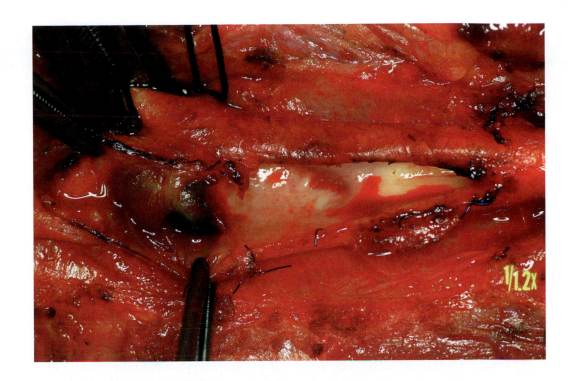

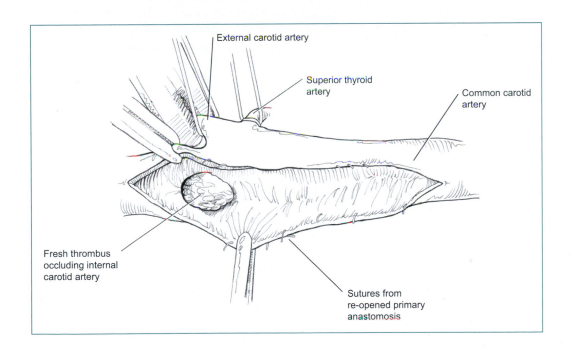

External carotid artery

Superior thyroid artery

Common carotid artery

Fresh thrombus occluding internal carotid artery

Sutures from re-opened primary anastomosis

4-2

Technique for Exploration of Complete Carotid Occlusion

It may be necessary to explore a complete carotid occlusion by virtue of a postoperative thrombosis or encountering a patient who has acute thrombosis of the carotid artery for other reasons and who happens to be in a position to undergo immediate surgery. When this situation arises, I perform the most gentle dissection possible of the carotid artery and cross-clamp only the common and external carotid arteries; the superior thyroid artery is isolated with a Potts tie in the usual fashion. No clamps are placed on the ICA since placement of a clamp in that location might dislodge thrombus and allow it to migrate cephalad. When the arteriotomy is performed, there should be no backbleeding because all sources of potential backbleeding have been controlled. I place gentle suction up the ICA first, but customarily this is ineffective in establishing backbleeding. My next preferred method is to attach a piece of shunt tubing to the end of a blunt needle and establish a vacuum system by connecting this to a syringe. The shunt tubing can be advanced up the ICA, as demonstrated in this illustration, until it encounters the thrombus, after which the syringe plunger can be drawn back to establish a vacuum. As this is withdrawn, it pulls the thrombus down into the operative field and copious backbleeding often follows. This procedure can be repeated several times, progressively pulling out more pieces of thrombus. Failing this, the technique of choice would be the placement of Fogarty catheters, which will be illustrated next.

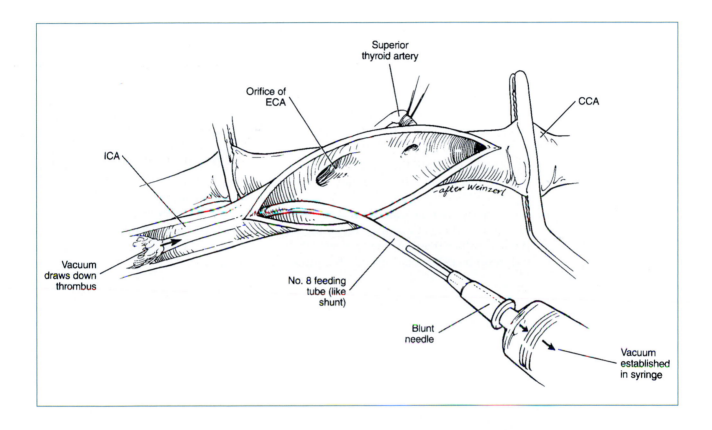

4-3

Use of Fogarty Catheters to Reopen Thrombosed Internal Carotid Artery

If satisfactory backbleeding is not obtained with the method previously described for thrombus removal with a shunt tubing on a blunt needle, a Fogarty catheter can be used instead. The problem with Fogarty catheters involves documented reports of the creation of a carotid cavernous fistula by inflating the balloon in the cavernous carotid artery. Nonetheless, if there is no other technique available to reestablish backbleeding, a Fogarty catheter is a useful choice. As shown in the illustration, it is advanced up into the region of thrombus. The balloon is then inflated and the catheter is withdrawn, pulling thrombus with it. It may be necessary to repeat this step several times before adequate backbleeding is obtained. It should be emphasized that copious backbleeding rather than a mere trickle should be the endpoint with either method and in the absence of significant backbleeding, it may be wiser to perform a stump ligation and closure of the ICA rather than settling for reestablishment of flow with an upstream thrombus that will then be catapulted up into the intracranial circulation.

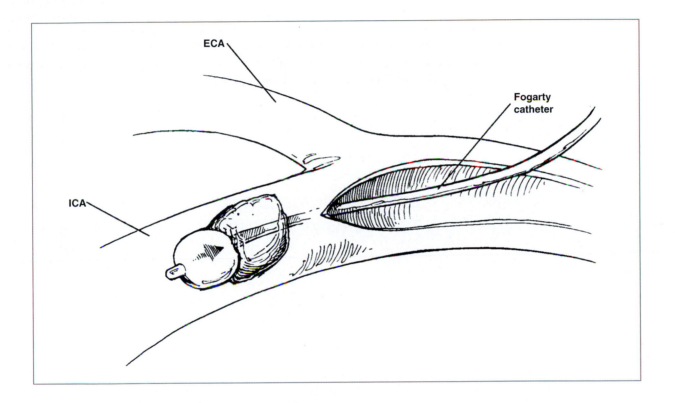

4-4

Postoperative Wound Hematoma

These two illustrations show an AP (A) and lateral view (B) of a patient who developed a postoperative wound hematoma on the first day. This particular patient had a prosthetic cardiac valve and was maintained on full heparinization postoperatively before being converted back to coumadin. He was neurologically intact and had no airway problems. We were concerned about an aneurysm, of course; however duplex scanning confirmed an intact carotid repair with no evident problems, and the hematoma resolved spontaneously without further issues. I feel strongly that a wound hematoma such as this needs to be investigated in some way to confirm the integrity of the repair, whether by duplex, MRA, CTA, or catheter angiography.

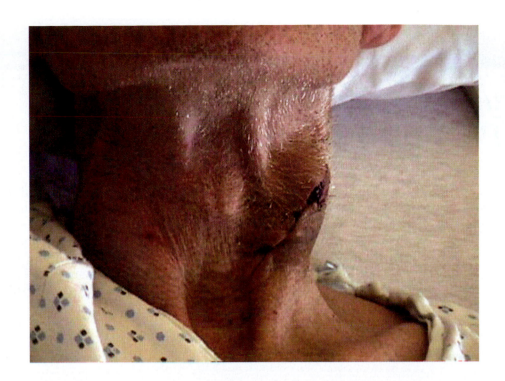

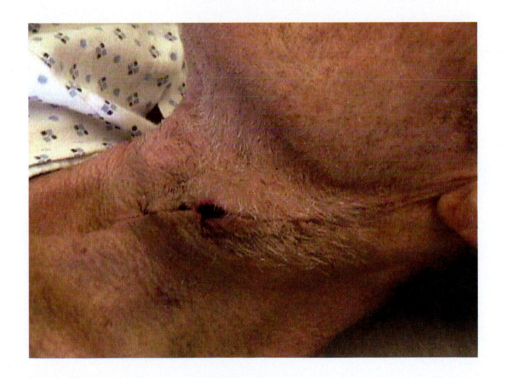

4-5

Aneurysm Formation Four Years Postoperatively

This case is of an older woman who had an uneventful left CEA with Hemashield roof patch four years prior to this event. She was neurologically intact. She presented to our ENT service with a neck mass (A) not related to any inciting event; specifically, she reported no trauma or heavy exertion, also no pain or bleeding. The radiologists read both her CT and MRI/MRA scans as being normal. Nonetheless, I was sufficiently concerned that I ordered catheter angiography (B), which demonstrated this aneurysmal segment along the repair. She was treated with a stent with good results, and the mass resolved with no complications of any kind.

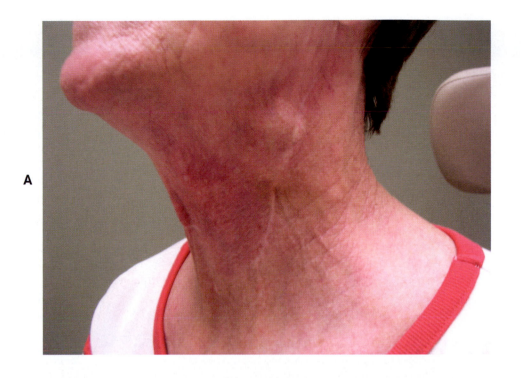

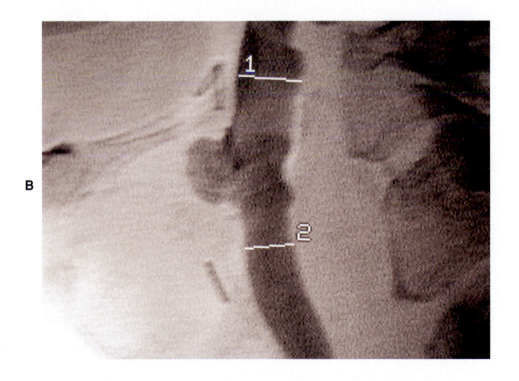

CHAPTER 5

Special Cases

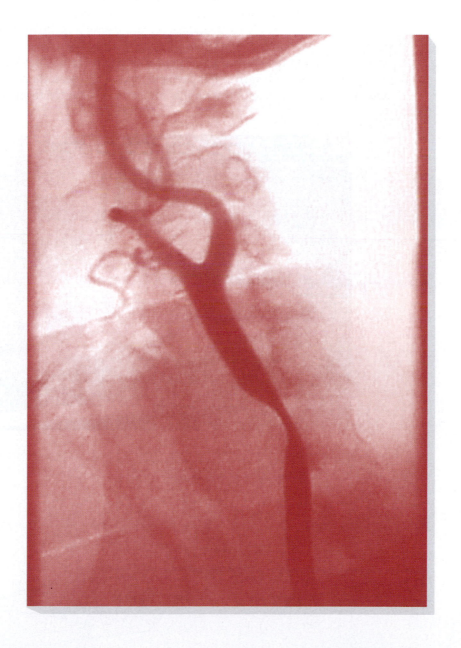

5-1

Treatment of Isolated Common Carotid Artery Stenosis

In this case a 56-year-old woman had stereotypic TIAs referable to the right brain and an isolated 70% stenosis in the right common carotid artery only. The carotid bulb and the external and internal carotid arteries were relatively free of disease. We made a decision to perform a purely CCA endarterectomy, which is illustrated here. In (A) the vessel is seen with the blue line drawn in preparation for arteriotomy. In (B) the artery is shown following uneventful repair and roof patch Hemashield graft placement.

An unusual case such as this demands special surgeon concentration on the clamping and declamping steps to be certain that the brain is protected from air or debris at all times.

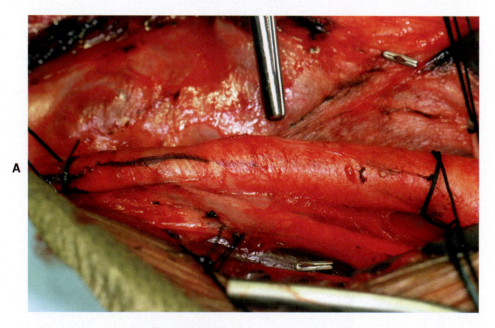

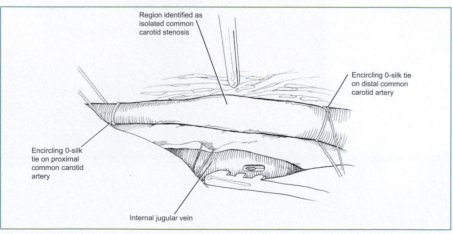

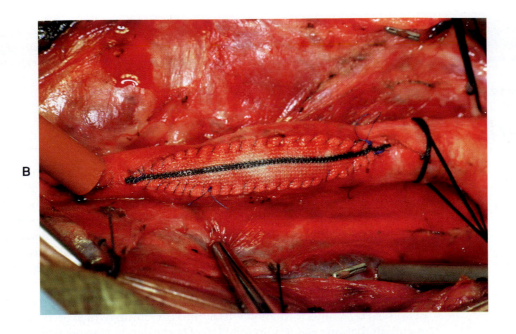

B

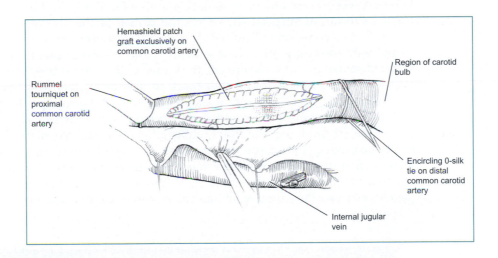

Hemashield patch
graft exclusively on
common carotid artery

Region of carotid
bulb

Rummel
tourniquet on
proximal
common carotid
artery

Encircling 0-silk
tie on distal
common carotid
artery

Internal jugular
vein

5-2

Treatment of "Stump" in an Occluded Internal Carotid Artery

The "stump" syndrome, as described previously in the text and illustrated in Figure 2-15, occurs when the internal carotid artery has occluded spontaneously, but distal to the carotid bulb, leaving a blind sac or stump. The stump may be small or quite large. TIAs can ensue when embolic material forms in the stump and embolizes up the ECA and into the cerebral circulation by trans-ophthalmic collateral pathways. I believe that symptomatic stumps should be surgically repaired, although the necessity to treat asymptomatic stumps is less clear.

In these four illustrations I show two such cases of stump repair. In (A) there is clear fresh thrombus formation within the ICA stump, which accounted for the breakoff of emboli that propagated up the ECA. This stump was oversewn and eliminated once the thrombus had been vacuumed away with suction (not shown). In (B, C, and D) I show a second case of a symptomatic stump as well, but in this case no fresh thrombus was found at surgery. (B) shows the orifice of the stump (empty in this case) exposed via a common to external carotid endarterectomy. (C) shows this stump sewn closed with interrupted 6-0 double-armed Prolene sutures placed from the inside out and tied so that the knots lie outside the lumen of the carotid tree (like a tacking suture). (D) shows the placement of a roof patch to maximize flow from the common to the external carotid, and the securing and obliteration of the stump with a large Weck clip across the base of the ICA (in addition to the oversewing step).

Some surgeons feel that simple obliteration of the stump externally with a Weck clip or silk tie is adequate, and do not open the vessel at all. I think this is dangerous for two reasons; first, that a clip applied externally to a flowing vessel could dislodge embolic material into the ECA and thus to the brain; and second, that an external clip does not completely obliterate the stump as an internal exposure and oversewing step will do.

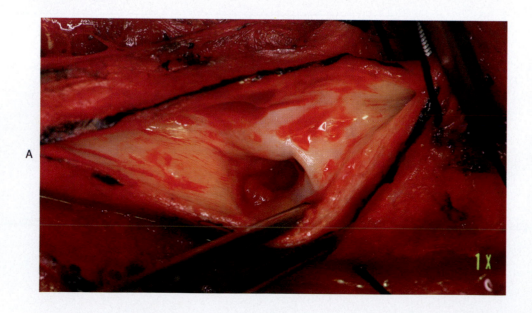

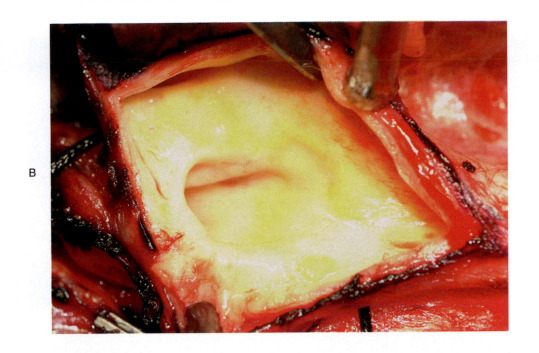

B

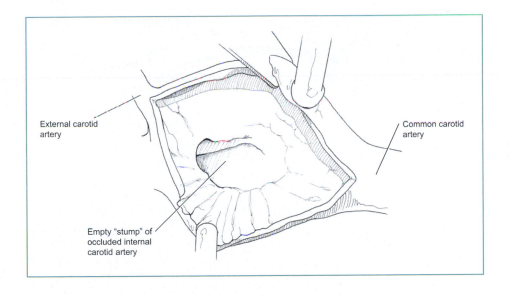

External carotid
artery

Common carotid
artery

Empty "stump" of
occluded internal
carotid artery

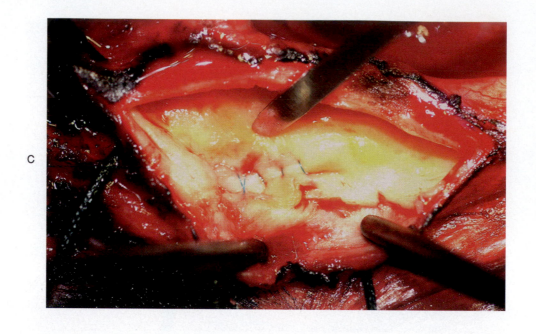

C

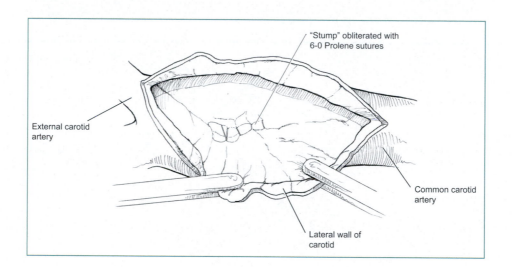

"Stump" obliterated with
6-0 Prolene sutures

External carotid
artery

Common carotid
artery

Lateral wall of
carotid

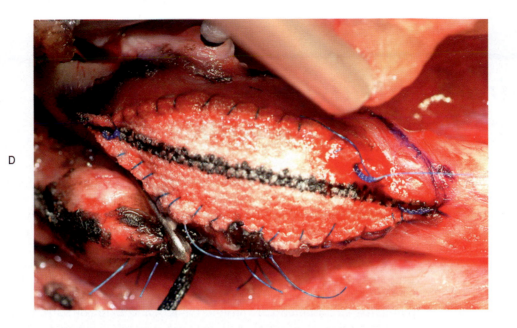

D

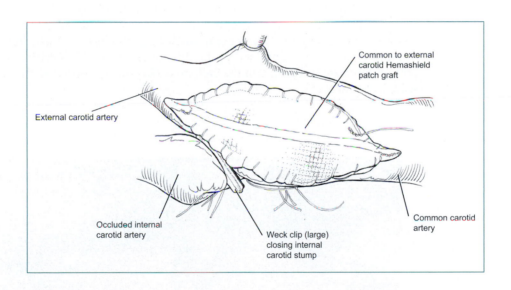

External carotid artery

Occluded internal carotid artery

Weck clip (large) closing internal carotid stump

Common to external carotid Hemashield patch graft

Common carotid artery

5-3

Repair and Straightening of a Large Left Carotid Kink

This patient had a right cavernous carotid aneurysm that was scheduled for endovascular balloon sacrifice of the proximal carotid. At angiography she was found to have a significant, flow-limiting kink in the left ICA. Both the patient and the interventional radiologist requested that this kink be surgically reconstructed to maximize flow prior to her carotid sacrifice.

The surgical procedure is shown in (A) and (B). In (A), the carotid tree has been completely dissected out and the double kink is easily seen in the ICA. The dissection needed to be much more extensive than a routine endarterectomy because of the need to mobilize circumferentially around the ICA and to uncoil/unravel the kink.

Once this was accomplished, the next question was how to best maintain the vessel in the unkinked state. One choice would have been shortening the vessel with an end-to-end ICA anastomosis. I chose, however, to place a Hemashield roof patch to stiffen and straighten the vessel, and then I anchored both sides to the surrounding soft tissues with 6-0 Prolene "angiopexy" anchoring stitches, as illustrated in (B). The postoperative angiogram, obtained at the time of right carotid sacrifice, showed a straight and widely patent repair, and the balloon occlusion proceeded without incident or neurological events.

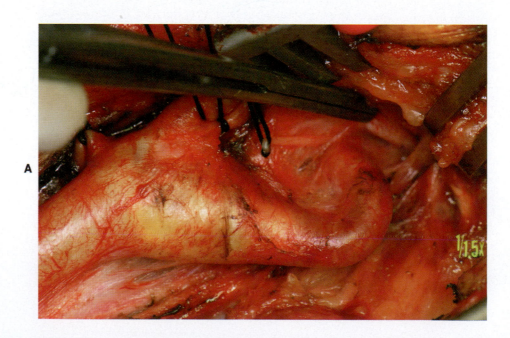

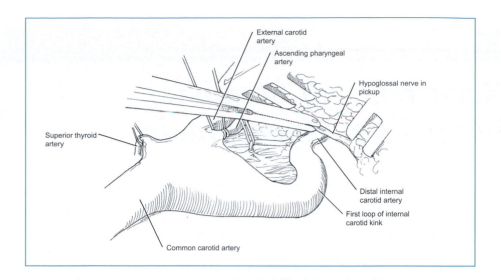

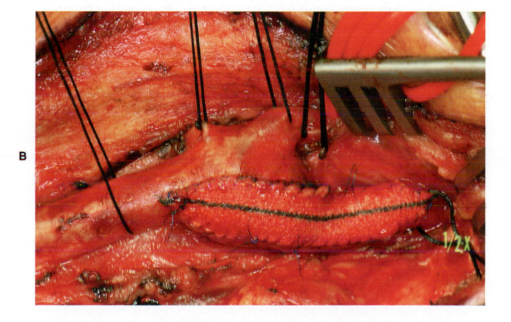

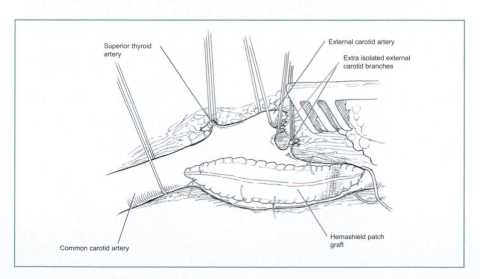

5-4

Rapid Recurrence of Stenosis from Myointimal Hyperplasia

There are two main causes of recurrent stenosis, aside from technical error. These are myointimal hyperplasia, which is usually rapid in onset, and recurrent atheromatous disease, which takes longer to develop. In the case illustrated here, a 45-year-old man with familial hyperlipidemia was operated by me with an 80% asymptomatic stenosis without a patch graft (this is an older case of mine). He returned six months later with routine duplex scans that showed a rapid recurrence (90% stenosis), and he chose to be re-operated with a roof patch (in this case a saphenous vein patch) as I recommended to him. At surgery we found a thickened fibrotic vessel wall with no real evidence of atheroma. A plane was developed with some difficulty and an uneventful patch graft repair was performed, after which he did well in long-term follow-up, with no late evidence of recurrence.

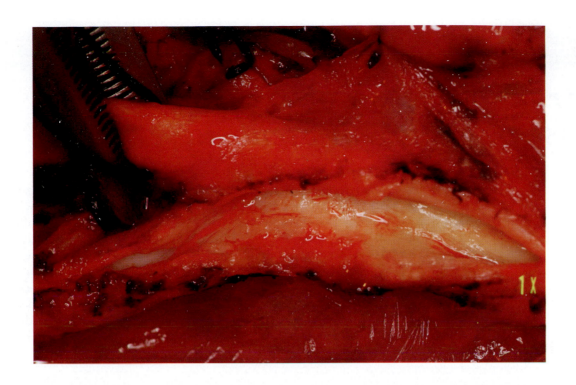

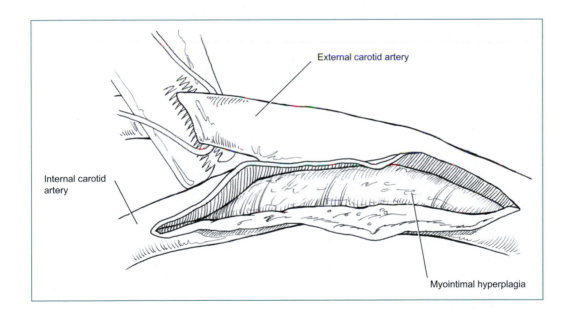

External carotid artery

Internal carotid artery

Myointimal hyperplagia

5-5

Scarring in the Carotid Sheath in a Case of Recurrent Stenosis

An operation for recurrent stenosis is significantly more difficult than a primary endarterectomy because of the inevitable scarring in the carotid sheath, which distorts the normal anatomy and obscures the usual tissue planes of dissection. I illustrate here an example of recurrent stenosis. The principle in this surgery is to identify the CCA as quickly as possible and dissect up directly over the vessel wall to obtain the requisite exposure. The vascular pickups in this photograph are holding up the tough scar tissue that overlies the common carotid, and one can appreciate the plane underneath this which should be blunt/sharp dissected with the Metzenbaum scissors. The positions of the jugular vein and vagus and hypoglossal nerves may be distorted, and in my experience the best way to avoid damage to adjacent structures is to stay close to the artery and peel all other tissues gently away from it.

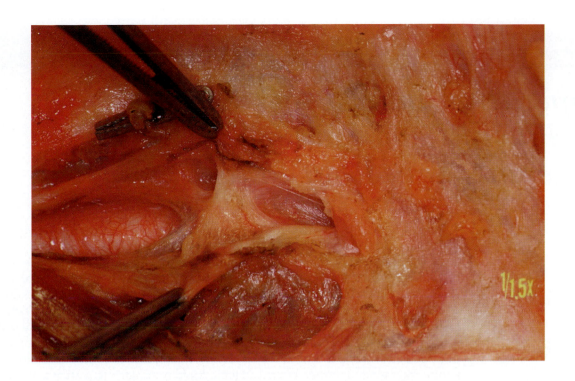

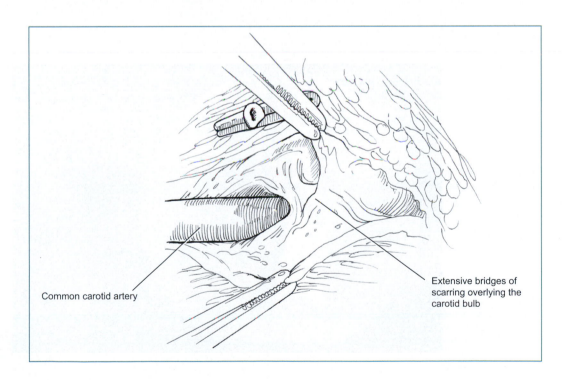

Common carotid artery

Extensive bridges of
scarring overlying the
carotid bulb

5-6

Reoperation in a Case Previously Repaired with a Saphenous Vein Roof Patch

This patient was presented to me by our neurology service fully heparinized with crescendo TIAs and recurrent stenosis, two years after repair elsewhere with a saphenous vein roof patch. In (A), the lateral angiogram showed tight stenosis in the distal ICA. I approached the case with caution, concerned that we would encounter a thin, friable vessel wall with a high likelihood of premature bleeding. The clinical situation was quite different than I had anticipated. (B) shows that the vein patch had actually completely endothelialized and was firm, thick, and easily dissected. The only real way we could tell which was vein and which was native vessel was from the old Prolene suture line. We performed a routine endarterectomy, taking care of course to remove all the old suture fragments, and then placed a Hemashield roof patch (C), after which the patient had a routine and uncomplicated postoperative course.

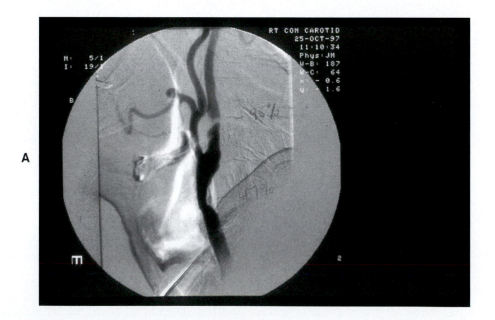

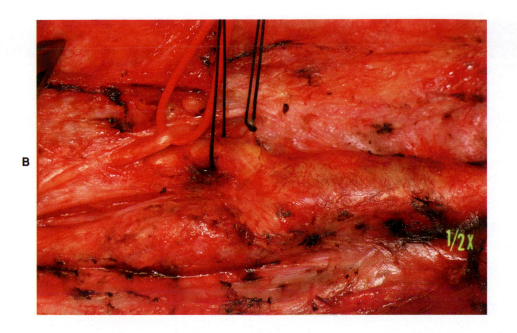

B

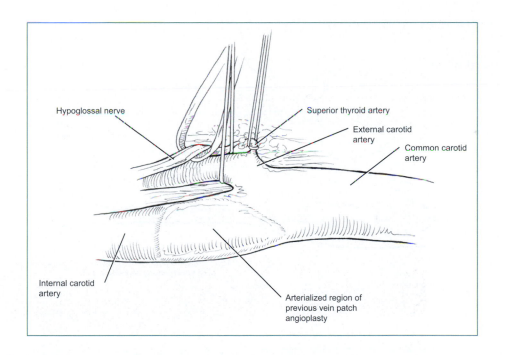

Hypoglossal nerve

Superior thyroid artery

External carotid artery

Common carotid artery

Internal carotid artery

Arterialized region of previous vein patch angioplasty

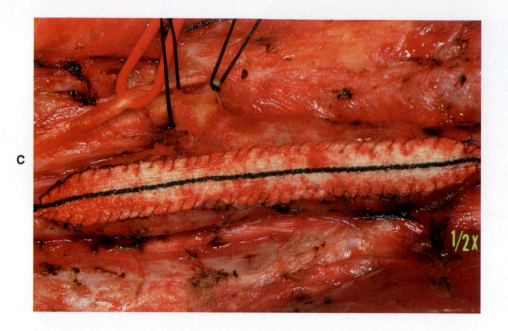

C

1/2X

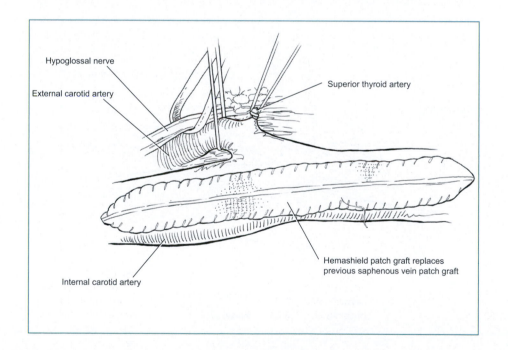

Hypoglossal nerve

External carotid artery

Superior thyroid artery

Internal carotid artery

Hemashield patch graft replaces
previous saphenous vein patch graft

Index